HOW
TO BE
BRAVE

Emilia Adler

Grosvenor House
Publishing Limited

This book is published by
Grosvenor House Publishing Ltd
Link House
140 The Broadway, Tolworth, Surrey, KT6 7HT.
www.grosvenorhousepublishing.co.uk

A CIP record for this book
is available from the British Library

ISBN 978-1-83975-367-1

To *the friends who showed me what friendship is.*

To *the strangers that smile on the street.*

To *P, for everything she's done.*

To *my family who never gave up.*

To *J, who is helping me come back to life.*

To *R, for being you.*

To *the brave person reading this who needs a little bit of hope.*

I wouldn't call myself brave. It's hard to say that about myself when I feel I've been so weak. I think you'd say that about yourself too. It's not everyday someone asks you to describe yourself and you say 'I'm brave'. But actually, we all are, we are all so incredibly brave.

For anyone who needs to hear this, I know life can get a little bit messy sometimes, but I hope I can help you even just a little bit to untangle yourself. I have always fantasised about writing my own book, and now it feels right, because I need to find myself and let out everything I've been wanting to scream to the world over the past few years. For me, writing is my way of finding out how I feel, what I'm scared of and who I really am. I'm going to say this from the beginning, I am not a professional, just a teenager with a lot to write about. My experiences have been my lessons, and that is therefore the most real thing you could possibly read. Some parts may also be triggering or upsetting, so please be aware of that. I hope the rest of the book brings you happiness and helps you find yourself. I also want you to know this: I have battled with my mental health for over 4 years now, and so much has happened. I can't reduce all of the events that have happened into a book. It is bigger than I can ever fully project, but I will try my very best. I hope you finish this book with understanding and a bit more hope.

I was born,

I died,

I was born again.

The storm cleared my path to start a new life,

Away from the painful memories of the past.

I've been blessed with another chance at life,

And I refuse to waste it

I choose to heal this time
I choose to grow and find myself,
For I've been lost for too long.
It's time to be happy,
It's time to be alive.'
Falling down is a part of life. Getting back up is living.

A lot of my life has been spent trying to shrink myself. Torturing my mind. I've always wanted to be liked, to be wanted, to be needed. I felt unwanted and unnecessary and stupid at school. I was 'that' girl. The girl who was always early for her lessons. The girl who always did her homework and wasn't 'naughty'. I was the shy one. The one who hated speaking in front of the class and doing presentations. I was the quiet girl. I'd wait in a classroom sitting alone on my table as the rest of the class bundled up in a circle and laughed until the teacher came. I just didn't fit in...I was always the outsider who would rather do sudoku (my favourite) than decide which photo is better. My anxiety was increasing a lot because of this. And so, I needed control. It became a habit. Soon after that during lunch times I would reduce my intake and just make a joke or lie out of it saying I had a huge breakfast or wasn't feeling hungry. What I want you to understand is that it was never about wanting to be skinny like models, it was about wanting to take up as little space in the world as possible because I felt so weird anyway. I did not develop an eating disorder because of the media, but because I hated my life. It wasn't about hating my body; it was about hating myself. I felt so out of control with things going on in my life that cutting and food became my control. But the thing is, it isn't just your body that shrinks. You get smaller, but so does your will to live, the size of your heart and the function of it. Yes, you're fading away, but so is your smile and laugh that used to bring happiness to so many people. Yes, you are dying, and the people around you are watching this disorder tear you apart, later by layer, bit by bit. So really, while you get smaller, your chances of death increase and your time on earth decreases.

I can't explain what it feels like to be suffering in that way. I can't tell you how it felt to be more scared of an apple than dying. I remember the nights when I couldn't sleep alone and my pulse was being checked every half an hour. I would sit down and my chest would hurt and feel heavy. There was a point where I wouldn't even leave my room for 2 weeks, I even brushed my teeth in my bedroom. I had no energy or motivation for anything, I was just completely out of it, possessed by this horrid disorder and dark thoughts. The room would move around me, even I would float sometimes. I was not myself. Not one bit myself. There have been moments where I have been really close to the edge, really close, falling down heavily. There are still days where I shock myself that I'm alive, and I guess that's also why I'm writing this book. I've seen how short life is, and I know that I will regret not doing this, because I have so much to share, and I need to get my words out. Most books like this are written by those who are recovered and thriving in life, but I want to be really real with you and write this as a teenager who is still recovering, being fully honest with you about life, recovery and society.

My biggest turning point was when I got sectioned in 2019 for the second time (I first came into contact with services in 2016) and was finally forced to gain weight properly and get to a healthier place mentally. Once I was discharged, my goal was, and still is, to be happy, live well and work on myself.

I want to also quickly say a huge thank you to anyone who has been with me along my journey, whether it's my Instagram followers, professionals, family, friends or even the lovely shop keepers. I don't say this enough, but thank you, and I am so sorry for turning your lives upside down and hurting you. I'm sorry I haven't shown you much love, it's just been hard to, because how can I give you my love when I don't even know how to love myself? You have all been so good to me, and I love you so much. I'm sorry if you've seen me hurt myself, in a terrible state, or if I didn't let you even come near me. I'm sorry if I let go of you even when you were holding me, wanting to be there. I couldn't face people to see me the way I was, because the truth is, I had lost the will to fight. And I wanted you to remember me as the girl full of life and happiness, not as a sick girl who had forgotten how to smile and laugh. I wanted your last memory of me to be a good one, I was trying to protect you. Please forgive me, I am sorry. But I am coming back now; you're getting me back. The girl with a bright smile and glistening eyes...she's coming back to all of you. Hold on, I'm on my journey home.

Emilia x

Book not recommended for under 15 years old.

PART ONE

My story

My Story, life growing up

"I still think my thighs are too big. And sometimes my sadness is overwhelming and I want to stay in bed. But I don't. I wake up and eat my breakfast. I eat food that I actually like instead of food with the least number of calories. I speak my thoughts and feel my feelings and get on with my day. I still need help. Some days I think about not eating. Some days I cry because my clothes are tight. But I bought new clothes, really nice ones that look great. I don't have a gap between my thighs, but I have legs that walk me around beautiful cities. I am living a life I choose, because I choose to live."

I was born at 1.50pm on the 23rd of April, as a happy and healthy baby who came into this world with many people already loving me. My life growing up was actually pretty great, it had its ups and downs of course, but all in all, I think my childhood was really good. I have memories of going to the park every day, no matter the weather, and playing barbies or shopkeepers with my mum for hours. However, by the time I'd gotten the shop set up I was too tired to actually play anymore. I remember my dad would take me to see aeroplanes at the local aerodrome. We'd just sit on the grass next to the runway with an ice cream in our hands...and our faces, and we'd just watch the planes 'magically' take off and land. My brother was always protective of me, and photos of him and me show such a huge bond of sibling-hood. I'm fortunate enough to have amazing grandparents, cousins, aunts and uncles. I'd go shopping with my grandma, we'd go to the park, the theatre, we'd bake and read 20 books consecutively. One of my grandma's had to put up with my teaching. I was taking my role very seriously, and she had a proper folder, pencil case and exercise book. She'd answer the register, and we'd get on with class. According to her I was quite a strict teacher, which makes me cringe at my younger self. In my spare time I'd type out maths exams, make up stories for a comprehension and so on. There was a point where I was even giving her homework. – I feel so embarrassed writing this but I'm pleased she played along and was the perfect pupil for me. We did, at one point, even attempt Finnish lessons, but I think we gave up a week or two later...there was no chance of her learning it. My grandpa would show me how to fish, how to cut down trees, how to light a fire and cook sausages over it in the middle of a forest and how to change a lightbulb. Even after sharing all of my 'beautiful' drawings of my family that I did as a child, with completely disproportionate body parts, they always smiled and said they thought it was the best thing they'd ever seen.

I've lived in the same town my whole life, and it's been lovely, and has made me feel safe. It has definitely changed over the years, but I don't think I ever want to move away, it's my home. I love going to the shops and knowing the workers, I love walking down old lanes that I used have toddler classes in. I've grown up lucky in a kind household where there was always a home-cooked dinner on the table, and exciting summer holiday adventures around the world. I'd see my parents every day and we had the opportunity to go out and explore the world. I've felt loved my whole life, and I know not everyone has had a life like that growing up, so for that I am grateful.

I was always the shy child, but people told my mum that I would grow out of it. I hated sleepovers, at dinner parties I'd much rather have sat on my mum's lap and colour, listening to the 'grown up conversation' than going off and playing with other children and would never say hi to strangers, but would instead bury my head in my mum's arms. I had an attempt of a sleepover at around 7 years old with a family I knew very well, which ended at 11pm when I had to be picked up in tears because as I was walking to the toilet, I saw a black phone on the stairs and screamed, thinking it was a mouse. I've always been a bit 'funny' about a few things. I'd hide my best toys when someone would come over because I didn't want them to be changed or ruined. I'd spend hours finding something to wear, and I never ever wore jeans. I was pretty well behaved, and *had* to follow rules. I listened so carefully that I never got anything wrong. I was a quiet, reserved child. For a few years I was doing Speech and Drama, and one year at the local arts festival my group was meant to recite a poem, 'Bella had an Umbrella'. Typical me of course had to first spend time crying under the chair and clinging onto it whilst my mum was trying to pull me up. Eventually I got up to the stage with a snotty nose, an angry face, and I just stood there with my purple umbrella, clearly not impressed. At the end of term ballet performances, I refused to let my mum watch me. She once peeked out of the door but once I noticed that and let her know, and probably let everyone else know, she was never sneaky again. I've definitely always been stubborn, but always been kind. I don't like certain foods touching each other, I don't like sitting on seats on public transport that have just been sat on, and my sense of humour has always been a bit different to others. In year 1 we had 'joke time', in which we all took turns to tell the class a joke. Of course, like all other 6-year olds there were the general jokes like why did the sheep cross the road. Then it was my turn... what a disaster. My joke involved a burning house, dogs, firemen, an essay of an explanation...and even though I found it hilarious I don't think anyone else did. I think that was the beginning of a big realisation that my sense of humour is completely different to everyone else's. Looking back, I realise that a lot of things I faced were sensory related, but as a child, it was easier to get away with picky eating and wanting to be with my mum. It's only now as a teenager when the struggles have appeared more. For example, I can't touch the sink, the rubbish bin or make my own bed. As a 5-year-old, I wouldn't have had to do these things so we didn't see it as a problem, but at this age I should be making my own bed and washing up, and putting my rubbish away. But I can't, I really can't.

When I was one, I learnt to walk. When I was two, I started to talk. By three I was a ballerina, and at four I could count to 20. At five I was in love with Peppa Pig.

At six id learnt my manners. At seven my friends were my world, and by eight I'd swum half my life. at nine I learnt about the world, the good, the bad and everything I between. When I was ten, I had everything I needed. When I was eleven, I was happy and completely alive. Then at twelve I learnt to scratch my anxiety away. At thirteen the world turned dark. At fourteen I was lonely, so a friend made a home in my mind. The only thing is, it was all a lie. She turned out to be called anorexia. At fifteen I felt dead. That year I was also saved. Now at sixteen I feel like I need to let out all of the words I've gathered up over the years, for I've learnt a lot about life. The good, the bad and everything in between.

I had friends, lovely friends that I cared about a lot. I was never alone in the playground and was often laughing and skipping down the field. I think throughout my primary school years I must've gone to Disneyland with Justin Bieber 50 times, and married boys in our class so many times I'm surprised we didn't make it to the newspapers. I had my first playground kiss with a boy from my class in year 2 but I remember not enjoying it at all, definitely not as much as my friends watching us. My best friend and I were inseparable. We had one argument in the whole time of being at school, which lasted half an hour because we missed each other. Most years we would buy the same pencil case, and at lunch time's we'd give each other a bit of food from our lunchboxes, sneakily swapping the food under our desks. Me and her, we did everything together, on school trips we sat together, in assembly we sat together, birthday parties...everything. I even had a birthday party with just her invited! In PE when we did cross country in the summer, we'd end up behind everyone else because we were so focused on our conversations rather than actually running. We'd have play dates often and we usually always watched some kind of film, either our school plays, laughing at how silly we look, or something completely random. We'd play hospitals and do artwork and just have the best time. She was my closest friend, and I still can't believe just how close we were, and I'm so lucky to have had her. Along my journey, like with many people, some of them have left my life, but they will never leave my heart. A few of my childhood friends still keep in touch with me, but we are going our own ways, and that's okay. In reception I managed to get a school play role as an alien, and I even got my face painted green, which resembled how sick I felt with nerves. In year 1 I was a snowman who clearly forgot the dance moves...the DVD (yes, in those days we still had those large black DVDs) showed me having a little fail messing up my dance moves. I was so embarrassed and hot I'm surprised I didn't melt! Or on the other hand I'm surprised I didn't freeze! My already very pale face had to be painted white to cover up the bright red face I had on stage. Following on from my great roles, I became lead fire dancer in year 3. My bright red bob wig matched the colour of my face, and I sometimes think that that's why I got the role of lead dancer. I always used to go extremely red, and still do. I've been called a red shiny Christmas tree bauble and Rudolph's nose...very flattering. Finally, in year 6 I got two parts as something a bit daintier and cuter, a fairy and a mermaid. Oh, I was absolutely in love with my realistic mermaid costume and my fairy outfit. After having some embarrassing, funny roles, this was my time to shine...and I think I finally did, 'swimming' onto the stage with a pink wig and mermaid tail.

My biggest dream was to be a ballerina or a teacher...or both. I was probably one of the biggest Peppa Pig fans (unfortunately Peppa Pig World didn't exist then), I loved art, dancing, playing in the park and anything to do with Barbies. Dolls were a huge part of my life; I was obsessed with being their mum and I really treated them as actual humans. Writing was important to me too, I've documented so many little details growing up and saved pieces of paper and receipts from 2010, even snack wrappers from when I was 6. Writing has been my escape for a long time, and journaling things so that when I look back, I can remember every detail. I think I'll share this lovely account I wrote on 8.03.15. 'Dear reader, whoever finds this, I am born in 2004. What is your industry like? My industry was fabulous. I guess you're already living on the moon now and having flying cars. I hope you write a letter like me to the future and read this thoroughly. Best wishes, Emilia Age 10'. As much as I loved writing, I also loved reading. From the moment I was born, I was always read to, and a day didn't go by without at least 3 books being read. I think that got me into reading, and also, I enjoyed the escape. My love of reading has stayed with me all my life, and I go through them so fast I can't even begin to guess how many books I've actually gone through in my lifetime. I know that nowadays you can read books online, but that's really not for me. There is something beautiful about holding a book, feeling the pages, turning them and smelling them. My absolutely favourite book shop is the old Waterstones in London. It is so big I could just get lost in there, in the calm and peacefulness, and the most amazing smell. I also loved moving my body and being active. I would dance around the house and follow along children's programmes, I'd run around, jump on the trampoline, hula hoop, skip, or literally just spin around. My main sports growing up were swimming and dance. I started both of these at the age of 3 and loved them. I swum for 8 years and danced for 11, and the decision to stop in my opinion was the correct one. I used to pretend I was a swimming instructor with my mum, and in the playground, I'd do little 'circuits' for my friends pretending to be a PE teacher. The older I've gotten the more I have an interest in not just the sport itself, but the biology behind it, nutrition, anatomy and that kind of thing. I can't forget about my love for facts, numbers and statistics. Did you know otters sleep holding hands? Or that golf was invented in Scotland? Or that the national animal of Scotland is a unicorn? (yes, I know, a bit of a random one that is). I absolutely love documentaries, and I've seen most of the ones Stacey Dooley and Louis Theroux have created. I think I've lost count of the number of crosswords, brain puzzles and fact books that I've gone through.

I'm pleased that I was born when I did, in 2004. I grew up without iPhones and all the technology that came after that. My favourite part about the Nokia brick was the snake game, it was such a treat to play it, and I actually miss it sometimes. I'm glad that my childhood was spent playing with sticks and dolls and wooden toys rather than electric games and tablets. I'm glad that instead of wearing child Adidas trainers I was wearing those really uncomfortable plastic princess slip on heels. Instead of wearing crop tops I wore pink and purple dresses with flowers and butterflies. I see children at restaurants watching Peppa Pig...when I was little, I coloured or brought a little ball to play with. I know that this is today's society and the norm for children, but part of me is quite sad that they're growing up too fast and not experiencing the old ways of childhood. I mean, I remember when black boards were still used in school...I don't think some children even know what they are nowadays.

Dear little Emilia, I'm sorry I haven't grown up the way you thought I would. I'm sorry my arms are now left scarred rather than covered with your favourite temporary tattoos. I'm sorry I've been so sad and horrible to myself. You never deserved a future like this. I know that your pure and gentle heart would forgive me. You would hold me now and plait my hair, humming the sweetest tune. Little Emilia, keep smiling, keep playing with your dolls, and keep covering your arms with butterflies and flowers.

You're probably thinking, where did it all go wrong? The truth is, I'm thinking that too, and that thought crosses my mind nearly every day. I don't have an answer to that, but I can only try and be a detective and piece things together as best as I can.

If I'm correct, things started in year 7 when I moved into a secondary school, where I also luckily made a very tight-knit group of friends who I still text quite regularly. We'd spend lunchtimes laughing until we could barely breathe whilst also doing homework – we became pros at multitasking. With this group of friends, we went on the best outings, once we even went to Brighton. That was such a lovely day and I felt so 'grown up'. We had the famous fish and chips by sea, walked to the pier and went to the funfair, where, yet again, I embarrassed myself. There was this one ride that looked quite scary but also very cool, so of course I had to try it. A friend ended up videoing me and all you can hear are my shrieks of fear...oops. That was probably one of my favourite days out, and we managed to fit so much into that one day. We also would go shopping together ad try on the 'ugly' clothes and see how good they looked on us, we went to the cinema, to each other's houses and sometimes out for lunch. I think I slightly regret some of the stupid things I did and cringe when I look back, like faking an ankle injury so I could get out of the 200m sprint on sports day (I put a bandage on my ankle and had a pretend limp just to make it look real), not forgetting Halloween when I got so scared outside, I ended up running down the road screaming...not embarrassing at all. We were also at that age where love, sex and relationships become slightly more significant in our conversations, and those chats never failed to bring out a few proper belly laughs. I didn't have a lot of friends, but the ones that I did have were the best people I could ever ask for, and were real and true friends. Until writing this book, I thought year 7 was not too bad, but my detective work suggests otherwise. On the 2nd November 2016 I wrote: I hate the stares I get; I hate feeling ugly, and I'm writing this with tears in my eyes. My anxiety was increasing and by the end of year 7 and the beginning of year 8 I was very nervous. I would get stressed about speaking in front of the class, being picked on by the teacher, my hair looking weird, performing to the class and things like that. I was almost in constant state of worry, which I now understand was taking its toll on me. There were always those awkward moments when a teacher would say 'so, who hasn't said anything yet?', and everyone looks at you (i.e. me). If we were reading a book in English and we'd 'snake' up the room changing at each paragraph, I'd spend most of the time counting through the paragraphs to find mine, praying it wouldn't be a long one. I don't think I was able to understand and fully realise how I was feeling and why I was feeling that. We were told everyone gets anxious, it is normal, and especially during the beginning of puberty things can be a bit difficult at times. So, that's what I thought, that it was normal to feel how I felt. *"A poem I wrote at school: I've decided to live in a cave. A dark, lonely and cold cave. A cave where nobody else can come in, a cave full of lost dreams and hope. A cave where only I can go. Because that darkness, is the darkness I have become. I've decided to live in a cave, because that is me. Dark, lonely and cold."* It was during this time that I first 'hurt myself'. It wasn't a lot, other than digging my nails into my skin under the desk at school during a stressful lesson, and nobody saw, and the redness would go after half an hour. I remember thinking how 'clever' I was, managing my anxiety and it not really affecting me. I thought I was a genius. At this time, I didn't even know that self-harm was a thing. We hadn't discussed it at school yet, and it was something I had never come across either. That slight digging into my skin was the start of a long journey of self-destruction. What was once my 'secret' and my clever way to manage, soon became a huge mistake and a terrible addiction. *"I'm so annoyed as I never seem to be happy anymore. My head is a dark place and I'm starting to think school isn't the only reason why I feel like this. I think there is another reason to why I feel so helpless all the time, but I just don't know what it is. School starts again next week and I am so scared and anxious, which doesn't help when I'm feeling low anyway."*

It was at the beginning of year 8 that my mood was dropping, but that was also around the time my period was starting, so it just made sense to relate it back to hormonal changes and developing. And even looking back now it made sense to think it was that, because there was nothing in my life that would've really taken it down the path of 'mental health issues'. I wasn't exactly thought of as someone who'd get depressed or develop an eating disorder. I was such a positive happy person and I was such a foodie. I absolutely loved food and had no issue surrounding it whatsoever (in fact I probably had a healthier relationship with my body and food at that point than most people my age), and was one of those people who could eat a very large amount and stay slim. As my childhood body was petite and tall, I did have comments growing up saying 'you look like a model' and so on, and although I'm sure it was meant as a compliment, I didn't take it that way and found comments like that unnecessary and a bit uncomfortable. In year 8 when my body was growing and changing into a larger body of a woman,

I guess I struggled a bit with change – I'm not great when it comes to change anyway. I don't think I personally had issues with myself either, but when I heard someone say 'look at the size of xyz' or 'I hate …' I thought I might as well look at myself in that way. Not because I thought something was wrong with me, but because thought it was normal. I didn't really know how to be a 'normal' teenage girl and fit in with the neurotypical standards, so I just followed others and followed their lead, so if they hate their thighs, perhaps it was normal for me to hate them too. I don't believe this started my disorder though, I really don't, but it may have been the start of talking negatively about myself and criticizing my body. *"Hi, life has gone down. Sometimes I enjoy life, but not so much anymore."* As these physical changes were happening, it was hard to remember my younger self. She was alive, happy, and so full of life. Her smile was genuine and her eyes glistened with hope. She had endless amounts of imagination and her little laugh radiated so much joy. Her quiet voice would never stop talking and she'd always leave a little bit of fairy dust wherever she went. She had a constant ray of light around her, she was beautiful and unafraid. No meal was too big and no mountain was too high to overcome. She was loved and she was loving. She was life, and deserved so much more than who I became.

Being mentally ill from a young age is strange, you grow up thinking that one day you'll finally be brave enough to die, or then the complete opposite, you'll wake up and be perfectly fine. Then before you know it, you're 18 and you're confused because you never thought you'd make it this far, but you're happy you're alive. But you also feel alone, and scared to be in a world you didn't think you'd be in anymore. Being depressed is being sad, but there's more to it than that. It's not being able to find yourself in the surrounding darkness, or being happy one moment and with a flick of a switch you can be sad again. Depression is not for people who want attention, you can't fake yourself into a serious mental illness. The quietest people have the loudest, most chaotic minds, and it is so hard to live with. *''I'm now on antidepressants and have been self-harm clean for 3 months! I think I'm developing signs of anorexia..."*

Also...if I ever talk about my past; it's not so that you can feel sorry for me, but so that you can understand why I am the way I am.

The first two days on Section 2

Previous to this admission, a few months back I'd been here for a 72-hour emergency stay. A diary entry leading up to this: 9th August, it's stupid. When you're not in a crisis anymore you are left alone. The Home Treatment Team left me today because I'm going on holiday. Oh yes, my eating disorder is suddenly going away because I'm going away for a couple of weeks. Its fine isn't it. because I'm fine. Better than fine according to them. I've changed. I don't smile anymore, my eyes are a bit darker, I'm a little bit more disturbed. I see things. Dark, black shadows. Everywhere. But like I said, I'm fine. They say I am good.

13.10.18

Yesterday the legal team came home and put me on a section 2. I've been put on a 1:1, meaning someone is with me at all times. I cannot believe this is real. This is what you hear about and think will never happen to you…until it does. Last night me and the others watched some tv which was nice and this morning we are watching a movie. I slept badly last night, it's scary here. I know I've been here once before, but I don't remember much of it. I feel really different here, like a misfit, not sick enough. Mum just came which was nice, but I'm not allowed outside the unit until I have had two meals.

If I eat them, then I can go home later. Lunch was really hard and I cried, but I managed and did it! Being on a section is usually a warning, but I guess there comes a point where you can't be given more warnings because it's too dangerous, and now I'm determined to be taken off it as soon as possible. When I'm recovered, I want to help and inspire other people who are struggling. Anorexia won't kill me; I'll kill it instead. I've spent too long hurting myself, it's time to save myself now. If I have the strength to hit rock bottom, then I have the strength to get back up.

I am also so grateful for my family and their support; I know not everyone has a good support system. Sometimes it may not seem that I am grateful for what people do for me, but I really am. I am forever thankful for those who haven't given up on me and loved me even during the times I haven't been very lovable.

I'm not on any medication anymore because it's dangerous for my body right now, but It may be an option later down the line. I'm in the quiet room right now, but it's not very quiet…everyone has decided to come here.

I find that being on 1:1 during the day is ok, but at night it is hard. But I understand why I am on it; at night I get too scared to be alone. I'm really struggling to get my head around the fact that I have an eating disorder. I still don't believe I have one, I don't see myself as having one. If you had asked me this a year ago and told me that I'd be in this position, I would have honestly just laughed.

I've just played an hour of card games with staff which was nice. It calmed me down and distracted me from the thought of dinner. I just want to get it over and done with. I find that waiting is almost as bad as the actual eating. What gets me through it though, is my mental reminders and affirmations. I don't want any more chest pains, heart palpitations, breathlessness and blood tests. No more of that. I want to be healthy and happy and love food how I used to. I've found that mantras and affirmations are really helpful, my favourite one being '*I am strong, I am brave, I am beautiful*'.

I'm sad, dinner didn't go well enough to go home. I'm feeling disappointed, but I will try again tomorrow. I have cried so much today my head is so sore. Goodnight

14.10.18

This morning I feel sick, hot and sweaty. I'm too scared to tell my 1:1. My body aches and I feel dizzy. My knees, stomach, chest and head hurt, and my vision has gone blurry.

Good news! At 5pm I can go home for the night. As long as I eat, I can stay home. My heart rate this morning was 140 – no wonder I felt so sick. Lunch was an increase from yesterday, but I managed. I did it. I'm going home!

I ended up staying at home until discharge, still on section, coming to the unit daily just so they could see me. This was very confusing and all over the place, I didn't really know what was happening and I don't think I know now either.

Discharged 7 November 2018

Section 3, the turning point

Never forget that there is more fight left in you than you think.

I remember lying in bed with my heart thumping and my head pounding, knowing that I was vanishing. My lips were raw and cracked, my hands cold and blue. I didn't dare leave my room because who would want to see me with hungry eyes sitting at a table? My body was a battlefield, and my mind was where the casualties were. People became lost to a stranger, a girl with a mind that was a puppet, the disease being the strings. My disorder snatched my life away from me. It stripped me bare until hungry, ravenous eyes were left and a soul was starved. It broke me, it made me sick, shivering and hoping that the monster would just go. It felt as if it was killing me, leaving me crying for the pain and fear to go away. It distorted my thoughts, the worst being the question 'eat or die' and the answer being the latter. It took away my teenage years that I should've spent laughing, experiencing life and savouring the last bite of the meal on the beach. Instead, a once glistening spark had faded, leaving scars and memories that will never fully be gone from my mind, as they are printed over my body and this thing people call my soul.

This is also the time where I had already started my Instagram page. People often ask me why I share some parts of my life so publicly, and the simplest way for me to answer that is to say that I have this burning sensation in me that tells me this is what I need to do, that it is the right thing to do. Because I want people to know the raw, ugly truth. For me, it is not about likes or followers, it's about those butterflies in my stomach I get when someone send the most beautiful message. I want to mention a few positives about social media, since there's so much negativity surrounding it. Instagram is a blank page, and us users are the artist. If you choose to follow Instagram models and influencers, chances are you are going to feel bad. But Instagram isn't the one that is forcing you to look at these edited pictures or triggering things. A few years back when I went on Instagram my mood would always drop because all I could see was unrealistic bodies and all things to do with diet culture. It wasn't Instagram that made me follow them, it was me. Nobody forced me to click on diet pages and bikini model accounts. It was me who also decided to change. Now when I go on it, it's filled with positive messages, 'real' bodies and true happiness. Instead of feeling rubbish I actually feel better sometimes. I've realised it is my responsibility to use social media in a positive way, and now I have had no bad experiences for months. On that note, however, I still acknowledge that social media is very toxic for some people and can have serious consequences.

These are a few diary accounts from before I got sectioned.

Hard day, the illness won today. Really tough day, I ran away from therapy and they had to call the police. I feel so sick and weak, I am absolutely drenched in sweat and nearly vomited.

It is trapping me; my mind is a prison cell. I am dangerous and lonely. Day by day the voice of my disorder is getting louder and stronger, and I restrict. Then I binge. Then I restrict again, then I binge again. I have no control anymore; I just want to feel okay again. I can't stop myself from falling, I want to be beautiful.

I have this thing...called anorexia. Some people name her Ana. She's thin and tall, and seemed so nice at first. She told me she wanted to stay and be friends, and I let her. I've started eating less, and hating the girl I see in my reflection, and my life has become a mess. But Ana is still my best friend, I hope she always stays, because all my other friends have left. I hope she continues to keep me company, even though I'm scared. She never leaves my mind, and it's finally occurred to me that she wants me dead. I hate my friend called Ana because she's made my life hell. Please, someone hear my silent yells because she won't let me tell. Ana is my worst enemy, she's this demon, this devil in my body. She's imprisoned me, and I can't but do what she orders. I can't continue being brave.

I'm tired of living under this dark shadow, living in this hole. I need to save myself, and if I were to die tomorrow, I would not be satisfied with my life. I'd regret the missed dinners with family just because food was too scary. I'd regret all the times I took a blade to my skin just to try and numb the pain of life for a little while. I'd regret the days spent in hospital crying rather than outside living. I will never quite understand how I've ended up like this, but what I do know is that this isn't how my life will be forever. I'm obsessed.

With food, numbers...everything. I am so tired of drowning in my own thoughts.

WEEK 1, DAY 1-7

I don't really know much about my life at the moment. Lately it feels like I'm not really living, and I don't know how I'm feeling. I know the facts though, I'm sectioned, and this is no life. I need to let go, really let go, and start new.

The day I got sectioned, 29.4.19. I woke up that morning knowing that I had a home visit with my consultant, but little did I know, my life would be turned upside down. That morning was nothing out of the ordinary, although from the outside you'd have seen a fragile girl having something control her every movement. I remember looking out of my bedroom window, seeing her come out of her car, but then also noticing a few other smartly dressed people following her. Immediately I knew they were going to do a Mental Health Act Assessment, since I'd already had two before this. From the moment I realised that I had been lied to and kept in the dark, my mind just became full with rage. I was furious, and really struggled with unexpected situations anyway. I locked myself in my bathroom, and refused to even say hi to the doctors. About an hour later I heard heavy footsteps come up the stairs, and silent murmurs between them. My heart was pounding and I was squeezing my body tight, wishing they would go away and that this was all a dream. The knock on the door came, and I heard the words I had dreaded, 'Emilia, we are here to inform you that you are now detained under Section 3 of the mental act, and must immediately go to hospital. The ambulance is already here'. I remember that deep pit in my stomach I felt when I heard that, and although my mind was filled with tears, none would roll down my cheeks, instead the tears that would otherwise have come out from my eyes, filled up as an ocean in my mind, blurring reality, and washing my emotions, stripping me, leaving me bare as a cold, dying girl who was about to face the biggest fight of her life.

I froze, and refused to open the door, and so they forced their way in and took me down. I was threatened with being carried out by security, but managed to pull myself together just enough to get into the van, with blackened windows, and two security by my side. The 15-minute journey to the hospital was a painful, sad, and scary one.

I walked down the corridor in the unit and was taken to the quiet room, where I was sat down, and given my first snack. I remember that snack so clearly, a sticky, dried fruit granola bar. The rest of that day was filled with tears, blood tests, ECGs, physical observations, and loneliness. The next 3 days were spent alone in the quiet room, even my meals were eaten there. Occasionally someone would pop in and say hi or have a small chat, but otherwise I was left alone to come to terms with what was happening, and really process the situation. It was only on day 4 that I went to interact with the other patients.

I was still out of it on my first few days, so I'm afraid I can't tell you much about it, but all I can say, is that it was scary, and painful, and lonely, and tiring. My day was pretty much just waking up, going to the room where I'd spend the whole day, having staff with mee 6 hours a day as after every meal we must be watched for an hour. In those hours some staff would talk to me, whilst others just left me to get on with my scribbling and doodling. Those days were hard, and my routine got changed in an instant.

I do not pay attention to the world ending, for it has ended many times for me, and began again in the morning.

3.5.19

Last night was fun. Me and the other girls did our nails, and A painted mine! I feel so welcomed already, and It was so nice to just pamper ourselves for a while, especially since today has been a tougher day. I am starting to get to know some of the patients and staff a bit more now. I have school today which I'm slightly nervous about but I'm sure it'll be okay. I'm sad that the minimum time I'll be here is 6 weeks. I really want to go home and its only been 4 days.

Mum is going on holiday for a week next week and I don't know how I will manage it seems unbearable to know she won't visit me every day for a week.

If I can't exercise for a while, I think I will break. I need to move, not to please the disorder but to learn to be at peace with myself. It's tough here but it's the same for everyone else. I just need to try my best, and if I've survived years of pain, I can survive this. Also, I can't believe how slim G is, it's actually quite upsetting.

I just remembered I am not at school this afternoon; I have a big meeting. I just wish I have a discharge date but it's far too early to give one. Apparently, I have a checklist of things I need to achieve in order to be ready for discharge which I'm happy about as I can have a piece of paper with written points that I can look at for motivation.

My observations were just taken, so that includes blood sugar, blood pressure, heart rate, sats and temperature. We get weighed twice a week, on a Monday and Thursday, and occasionally spot weighed.

I've had a busy day today. The meeting was so pointless though. I hate my consultant I wish I didn't ever have to see her. But I know that one day this will all be a memory and I'll look back on this time of my life and be so proud I got through it. Right now, I feel disgusting and sick. This is awful. I am home sickness and want to exercise and breathe fresh air. I am struggling right now. I'm really jealous of those will leave, and they always come back with storied about what they did. I hope one day I will be that person. Fuck! Dinner was tough, but at least it was with S, one of my favourite staff members. A patient said 'even I couldn't eat that much' and that triggered me so much. That was the biggest meal I have had in months, even years. Thank goodness mum came after dinner and she lifted my spirits. she helped me shower, talked about her upcoming holiday and played connect 4. Then after she left A plaited my hair and we had such good chats with the nurses. My hair is so nice!

PS One of my rewards for getting discharged is me and mum are going Lanzarote in July. We can have fun and I can enjoy food and sit. We are also going on a cruise afterwards and I can really enjoy it because last year I was so caught up in my eating disorder that I couldn't enjoy it.

My friend once asked me what weight will be good enough. I replied that there isn't one, it will never be good enough. She responded saying, so you don't have one specific number? I whispered, I guess 0 anything. Her eyes opened wide and she said, you realise then that you wouldn't be living? I couldn't reply to that, so she asked me if it scared me. I had no answer to that either, so we just sat there in silence, motionless, the silence being the loudest answer of all.

4-5.5.19

Its Saturday! I don't know what's happening today as there's no school and it's the weekend. I find it hard to fall asleep here but when I do fall asleep, I don't wake up until morning. Day 5, let's beat this illness! Everyone is so proud of me as they thought I'd be screaming and making a fuss, but I haven't. yes, I've cried, but that is understandable. On the weekend we are allowed our phones the whole day which is good since there is literally nothing to do here.

Oh, my goodness they are messing with my meal plan. First, they gave me milk, and then a banana. I hate them and it took a lot of sorting out until they realised, I am allowed to say no to foods I actually dot like because of ASD. Normally the EDs are allowed 3 dislikes, but because I have sensory issues with food I am allowed to have more.

We're watching soap box races and it's so funny everyone is laughing! It was so nice to just watch it for an hour, comfortable on the sofa with patients and staff having a laugh. I'm writing a lot nowadays, and if I ever write a book, I will call it How to be Brave. Urgh I am so bored. Time goes by so slowly.

Mum and dad came and we sat in the courtyard it was amazing sitting outside for 15 minutes. I am feeling a lot more refreshed now. I had to get my observations done and my sugars were slightly low, so I guess lunch will help with that. I'm excited to see mum again later.

Just played the best game of Jenga it was so fun. Rumours are going round that a new girl is coming... and there is. She is here for a 72hour admission so just a short emergency stay. I'm not here to judge, but she is 13 and smokes and drinks often. I just find it sad how young she is and how she's harming herself and getting addicted so young.

Something I've found even in just five days of being here, is that patients become friends. Even for just 20 minutes we forget about being ill, and just get on with each other. We are living with each other and support and understand each other, I would never have crossed paths with some of the people here as we come from such different backgrounds. We are sharing such vulnerable times with each other and I already know I will never forget the people I have met. It's really hard to see someone struggling, but it's also so heart-warming to see sooner achieving their goals and doing well. I am proud to be a part of their recovery and their lives.

Yay great evening! Mum came again and we talked, cried and played games. Then after she left in the lounge the patients and staff were doing henna. C did mine so beautifully and G so kindly gifted me with a lovely stress toy. This was almost like a best friend night/ sleepover. A tiny bit of fun in a tough situation is always appreciated.

Morning! I'm really sad because today is the last day, I see mum as tomorrow she leaves for her week long holiday. Today I will make the most of the time I have with her. I actually slept pretty well last night. Today will be a bring day, weekend son the unit are just boring in general. Pretty much just meals, visits, and sitting on the sofa writing, colouring, reading, or watching tv or playing a game. The hours are very sow I have to say. Weight gain is awful but I'm managing. I love my henna though it's so pretty.

I've found a braveness and strength in me I never knew I had and being here has taught me to never take freedom for granted. At home you can go out when you want without a form saying you have permission to leave. You can shower and use the toilet when you want, unlike here you cannot. Once I'm free, I will wake up as go to bed with gratitude. I still have Lily's plaits! They have stayed so well, but I'm having a hair wash tonight so they will have to come out.

For over a year I have had no contact with people my age, so it's different, but nice to suddenly change to be living with so many people so closely, always around each other.

At the moment I am not in love with appearance. However, I am grateful for my body for keeping me alive even when I've hurt and fallen apart. I don't love my body for how it looks, but I love it for what it does for me. I hope to love myself soon, I'm working on it. I love my eyes so I can see the world. I love my ears so I can hear the most beautiful things. I love my legs for taking me wherever I want to go. I love my heart because despite everything, it is still beating.

Now watching Simpsons. Good old Simpsons. There's another new girl here, Eva. There is also good staff on today! I'm nervous as to when I will get my period back because I haven't had it for so long. I'm worried I will think getting my period back means I am fat, when in reality I know getting it back means I'm healthy and my body is starting to work again.

Before lunch dad came it was lovely to sit in the courtyard and play connect 4. Now I am actually so bored its tiring me out...I can barely keep my eyes open. They should really have some form of activity to do on the weekends. I still feel so lazy just sitting down all day long, but I'm plodding on. I miss home. I'm not sad or nervous today, just bored. 15 minutes seems like an hour, I really don't think I have ever experienced a level of boredom like this ever in my life. I definitely shouldn't be complaining at home on the weekends saying I am bored. Urgh so tired, this is unbearable I could just fall asleep right now. My eyes are all blurry and shut without me even realising. I haven't moved all day and my legs are so sore too. I think this is a cue to write something motivational so...I am ready to let anorexia go and let it go. I am ready to be me again, to really be me. People ask me how to be brave, and sometimes the only answer is 'tell yourself you are brave, then you are brave. I need to keep fighting. I have been sick for too long. I need to get better. No quasi recovery. No half recovery. From here my only way is up. From here there is no going back, no matter wat challenges I face. My past does not define me. my weight does not define me. I do not need to be the smallest person because it's not just my body that shrinks, its everything else around me.'

Just watched a bit of BGT which lifted the mood here, and got me slightly more awake.

Yay best time with mum. Hair wash and chat and she bought me 2 pens and a notebook as a present since she's leaving for a week. She also bought me new books and 7 letters for each day she is away. And afterwards my hair was plaited again!

6.5.19

You eat your cereal or cake or pasta even if that butch tells you otherwise. You tell her to shut up. To leave you alone. You're too busy for her. When she's finally gone there will a silence you have experienced for a long time. It will take time to get used to it. You may even miss her sometimes. But don't forget that she's trying to kill you and hurt you. Don't forget that you also have a life to live.

Good morning, I can't believe it's been a week since I was sectioned. In seven days, I have come really far. Last night was really noisy and I didn't get much sleep. I also hate how bright it is at night. Granny is going to visit me today. I am a bit nervous.

I've realised that colouring pretty much is one of the only things to do here that passes time. Most people colour, and its actually quite relaxing and distracting of what is going on.

Oh my goodness I am so happy. So happy. Me and a nurse went for a 20-minute walk in the fields I feel the best I have felt in so long. This feeling is indescribable. I have waited for a week to breathe real air and have a walk. Yay all my hard work this week has paid off. I am a happy girl now. I felt productive which is important to me. The rest of the afternoon I am writing, reading, watching tv and going on my phone. I can't believe I am writing this but I feel content. I am calm and satisfied. I even got to face time mum from her hotel. Then granny came and we played uno and had such a lovely time. Today has been good, goodnight.

CHAPTER 3, WEEK 2, DAY 8-13

7.5.19

7am weigh in was done. I have a CPA today.

For some reason my stomach hurts in a really weird way it's quite uncomfortable. Today is also ward round, it was nothing special. Ward round is weekly with the consultant, therapists, assistant therapist, a teacher from the school and other members of the team. I must say, at first it is quite intimidating walking into a room full of professionals staring at you, and sometimes it feels like you're on the hot seat, but I will get used to it.

My CPA went okay, again, nothing dramatic has changed. I'm really pleased though that I'm being taken off physical obs! Then I met with a movement psychotherapist, which is the weekly therapy I will be getting here. She seemed very lovely and I think I will enjoy working with her. I am grateful that my team have understood how hard talking therapy is, and that they've given me the opportunity to regulate my emotions through therapeutic movement. I have never even heard of this, but I am willing to give it a go!

Today has been quite challenging in terms of snacks, but I am proud of pushing through them and managing. Am I scared of weight gain? Yes. I am, I really am. But fighting through this Is the only way I will be allowed home.

Yay, after dinner, dad came and we went on a 45-minute walk and I face timed mum. It was so lovely to go out!

Goodnight

8.5.19

Yesterday was quite unsettled on the ward, so in the evening to lift our moods we played Jenga and had a lovely conversation. Yesterday people had many incidents and my meal plan was significantly increased. I'm hoping today is a better day.

Bang. The walls were vibrating. There was screaming. There was yelling. There were howls of pain and fear. Then silence. This was an everyday occurrence; I would soon find out. D, who was psychotic, was having an incident. All I could do was sit with the others, praying for it all to end. The silence of an IM was the end. But that silence would always speak louder than words.

The thing is, I think about dying often. But I really want to live. I don't want to die, not even close. In fact, I want to escape. I feel trapped and bored and tired. There is so much for me to see and so much for me to give but somehow, I'm glued in the same reality.

My goal is still to be out of here by the beginning of June. On a completely different note, my stomach still hurts. I don't feel great being here, I feel like being here is making me worse.

My day today was okay. School, snacks, meals...the usual. Same old routine. But I've kind of had a brain washing moment, where I believe I am worthy and enough. I have a bright future, and this is just a small mishap which will pass. This is a chapter of my life that will soon be closed. And that's brave, because I know that my best chance at freedom is to start a new chapter, even if my current one doesn't feel complete. Well... that's because anorexics wants the book to end, so... now I know what I need to do. And the best part about the new chapter is I can decide what will be written. I will begin it with me being in a healthy body and mind, really living.

It was as if the group therapist knew I was feeling motivational, we drew and wrote quotes! That was peaceful and motivating. This afternoon has actually been really good.

I think I spoke too soon; I feel awful now. Dinner was huge and so difficult. I feel awful. I really need mum and want to cry in her arms. I feel really sad now. Luckily granny came to play some good rounds of uno, it was a lovely distraction and made me feel better. After she left, I finished the day with more Jenga. I think by the time I'm out of here I will be a pro at it!

Goodnight

9.5.19

Morning weigh in. I'm a bit sad because I feel like I am at the perfect weight but I'm nowhere near so I'm scared I'm going to feel so fat and won't fit into my clothes anymore. I'm nervous as I don't know what I'll look like. I'll look so different to how I looked when I came in.

Normal day again today, except in school once a week they go to the gym at the local leisure centre and I'm not allowed to go which is sad. I just feel awful again. Tired, miserable, lazy and deflated. These past few days have been hard.

Just had my bloods taken! I have a huge fear of needles and blood tests and anything along those lines so I'm really proud.

A very kind patient is getting discharged today. I will miss her, but I am so proud of her and happy for her. We held a leaving tea party for her with cake and fruit, and it was a really positive energy. She made a great exit... there was the cake and also strawberries. She held up a strawberry for us all to see and said, 'what is this? I hate vegetables. She made the most iconic exit and left us all smiling. Seeing her has given me a bit more motivation as I know one day I will be in her position.

Then we had group therapy...I feel like a busy lady today! Afterwards to make things even better, my absolutely favourite staff P took me on a walk. I am so happy. (PS I think my mood is all over the place at the moment one moment I am so sad and then I'm happy).

To end my day mum's best friend came to visit me and we spent hours playing games which was so nice, she is amazing.

I feel positive, I've been productive today. Goodnight

10.5.19

Good morning, hoping for a good day. 3 days until mum is back yay!

Not much to write today, just school and meals which have been normal and okay. After school I had my weekly Friday group art therapy. There is me, 3 others and staff P and the art therapist. It's a really silent calming hour and at the end it actually gets quite emotional when we go around the table talking about our artwork and sharing personal thoughts and feelings. I even got to go on another walk with P. then dad came and I went on another walk. I feel really positive now.

I also thought I'd tell you a little bit about my room. Well, it's not a hotel room, it's extremely suicide-proof I must say. My door has no lock of course, and in the middle is a glass window that staff look through to see the room. In the room itself I have a very basic cupboard with no doors and one shelf, a wooden desk with a chair, a basic bedside table, and a bed. Of course, however, I have decorated it more to my taste...pictures, quotes, teddies and my own blanket. In my room I have my shower and toilet. The door however, is a bit different. Imagine a rectangle has 4 columns in it, that's the doorway. There is only a door in the middle two columns, meaning there is a pretty large gap between the top of the door and the bathroom, and the bottom of the door. This is obviously for safety reasons. To be really honest with you, I am not impressed with my bathroom. My little bum is put to sit on the little edge of the toilet seat – none of those 2 normal 'flappy' bits you get, one where you usually sit and the other the lid. I also have a mirror, a suicide mirror, I think. The reflection is a bit distorted, either because it is a safety mirror or then us ED's can't know what our bodies actually look like. I have a little sink with two buttons on the wall to get water. (they really do come up with everything). Now, the worst bit of all, and possibly quite funny, is the shower. It's this little, tiny shower head sticking out of the wall. Underneath it is another one of those buttons in the wall that you press. It's pretty much a lucky dip from there. Some rooms the water is freezing, some it's too hot. In some it runs for 7 seconds, some 30 seconds. You can probably begin to understand that showering is quite the performance, not forgetting the fact that the water sprays everywhere but on the body.

Goodnight

11.5.19

It's the weekend again, which means another slow and boring couple of days.

Some rules are so stupid. When I sit, I need to sit a certain way. Seriously? There's a right way for recovering anorexics to sit? I think it is ridiculous and uncomfortable. Imagine sitting down 11 hours a day and then sleeping at night. My backside is in agony and I have pins and needles. I don't understand why I can't stand up for 1 minute to stretch and shake my body just to make me less sore. I really do not understand this rule.

In between meals I have been colouring loads and was allowed to sit outside in the sun with some patients and staff.

Later on, dad and Daniel came and we went on a lovely walk and played some uno. Then just relaxing in the lounge watching tv.

Goodnight

12.5.19

Good morning. It's finally Sunday, and mum is coming back from her holiday!! I am so happy and excited.

After breakfast I've just been colouring, writing, watching tv and doing a bit of Jenga. After lunch dad came and we went on a lovely walk and it was so warm. Really good mood.

Mum came. Yay. So happy. We washed my hair and chatted.

Goodnight

WEEK 3 day 14-20

13.5.19

Happy Monday. I got weighed this morning, and for some odd reason I lost weight despite being really sedentary and being on a high meal plan. I'm going to prepare myself for a meal plan increase as that is what they're most likely going to do. I am so sad genuinely about losing weight as I was so sure I had gained and I was actually really hoping to. Urgh I am actually so annoyed. Tomorrow is ward round I hope it goes well.

It's really short-staffed today which is bad because there's not enough support. If I need the toilet, I sometimes need to wait over an hour...just to pass my urine. It's pretty shocking, I have to admit. When there's not enough staff things go all over the place and become stressful or unsettled.

Today has otherwise been ok, we had a group therapy which was fun, and then a nice short walk with P. I also saw mum and went for a walk with her which was lovely. We also played connect 4, and she gave me a gift from Cyprus which definitely put a smile on my face.

Goodnight

By the way there is the most disgusting ant infestation in our bedrooms. I feel like an animal, it's very unpleasant to have loads of ants everywhere, I feel so inhumane and gross.

14.5.19

'The world shines brighter with you in it. Maybe your own light has been switched off for a while but that doesn't mean the whole world is dark. As I trace the marks on my body is whisper "don't give up. You're more than your pain. You deserve better". Maybe life is full of rain right now, but image how many flowers are going to grow soon. If you're looking for a sign not to give up, this is it'.

Ward round today. Excited but nervous. I hope something good comes out of it, I have really tried hard.

Ok shit day. Absolutely rubbish. I had movement therapy and then ward round. Ward round was awful and so negative. I have no leave anymore and have been put on a 1:1...this is a nightmare. This is because I lost weight, and need to be on this level of observation until Thursday, when they'll weigh me again and take me off 1:1 if I have gained. I am so angry and frustrated. I was hoping for great news because I genuinely have tried so hard. Lunch was clearly an increase, but I just need to remember that this is another obstacle that I can overcome. I will prove to them and myself that nothing can break me. My current 1:1 is so lovely and is listening to me and talking with me outside which has calmed me down. Today did not go the way I had planned but I will pick myself up. Then my hair got plaited again!

Mum came which was so nice I had the best time. She really motivated me.

Goodnight

15.5.19

Morning. 1:1 overnight went okay. It's just very awkward and hard to sleep with the door open and someone constantly staring at you. what if I fart in my sleep? Or make noises? Or go into a funny position? And wake up with awful bed hair? Or need the toilet at night? Being on a 1:1 during the day is fine, no problem, it's the night time that is the issue. And using the toilet. Today's group was self-expression which was good. Mum came and I mainly cried, but had a few games of uno too. I also managed to have a shower. I'm glad I saw her, and hopefully tomorrow I am off 1:1. Ps a staff member who went on holiday bought us back bracelets! So, kind. Goodnight

I received a copy of my care plan today.

Here is my list of rules, goals and plans:

- I am to follow unit rules and be respectful
- I am to engage with the unit program and use therapeutic resources
- Before I go on leave, nurses will assess my wellbeing
- I am on a controlled meal plan and must comply with it
- Staff are to support and sit with me during meal times
- I am to attend school at the unit
- I am to engage with my treatment plan
- I am currently nursed on continuous supportive eyesight observations to monitor me
- If I become distressed or at risk to others, PRN should be given if verbal support has not worked
- If I have an incident, I must reflect with a staff
- I am to remain physically well
- I am to have regular blood tests
- My physical observations must be taken regularly
- I must allow my ankles to be checked for swelling
- Activity should be kept to a minimum
- I should remain seated with both feet on the ground, with my back on the back of the chair
- I need to rest as much as possible

16.5.19

Today I got weighed and I'm pretty sure I gained so hopefully...drum roll please...I get a bit of my freedom back!

Yay! I am off. My hard work has paid off and I've managed to get over another hurdle. I also had a great session about emotions with P which just made my day even better. I've also found out I am allowed a slow, snail paced 20 minutes' walk a day which is not a lot, but it is something, and I am grateful to be allowed that now. I feel deflated and rubbish though because I feel like I've gone backwards from over an hour of leave to 20 minutes. Mum came and it was nice to see her and get a bit of fresh air. We walked to the adult's hospital down the road and got my favourite, a Pepsi Max. What is even better is that it was a 20% bigger one. Oh, the joys of Pepsi max and how happy it can make me in the worst situations. Then back to the unit for some games with mum and some more colouring from her! I am so much happier this evening. And before bed a quick game of scrabble, perfect. I'll have a good sleep hopefully, goodnight

17.5.19

I can tell you it was bloody great sleeping without someone's eyes staring at my every move. Today is just an average day with more henna and nail painting! I also attempted plaiting a nurse's hair which was fun. I also had group art therapy which is one of my highlights of my week. Then mum came and we went on a 40-minute walk – yes, you read that right. In one day,

I've been upped from 20 minutes to 40. Yay! It was slow but absolutely amazing and so refreshing for my mind and soul. Today has been good, goodnight.

18.5.19

Its Saturday! Dad came and we played uno. Then mum came and I cried. And cried. Then dried my tears and went for a calming walk...and of course my Pepsi Max. I'm so lucky to have so many visits I am very grateful. I've had an ok day myself, but the unit is quite unsettled. To end my day granny came and we had our usual rounds of uno, and then a bit of tv in the lounge before bed. Goodnight.

19.5.19

Its Sunday and day 20. Almost another week gone. My goal for next week is to make more progress and get leave increased. Staff S, another one I get on with well has just given me such an inspirational and motivational speech. Dad came again, and you can guess, we played uno and had a walk. I'm quite bored otherwise today but getting through.

'They say that rain washes away the pain of yesterday. They say without the rain there would be no flowers. They water is cleansing and purifying, and the sound of water calms the soul. So, maybe the ocean of tears I cry are there to wash away my sadness and let a garden of beautiful flowers grow in me. Maybe the tears are there to purify me. Maybe tears are a sign of new life'.

Ok so this evening has been bloody tough. Mum came and I cried. Because I think it is completely natural to cry. I'm sectioned, in a psych unit, in a depressive environment, fighting my demons. I'd like to think everyone would cry in a situation like that, and it to be accepted. Well I thought so too. A nurse walked past the door and thinks I am having a tantrum. On top of that I'm moving rooms which I find hard so whilst mum Is sorting my stuff out, I am just in tears. Then when she was going to go, I got upset because she told me she wasn't going to come the next day even though I really need her. A staff member gets angry and starts calling me manipulate and abusive. He forces my mum out just like that. I feel awful, and trapped being locked away. All I did was cry and they made it seem like I was having a serious incident. I got threatened with an alarm being pulled and being restrained which in fact just made me even more furious. I feel ashamed for struggling and letting my emotions out.

I am forever grateful for the amazing patients here though. J and M came to hug me, and we had a little personal chat that made me feel a bit better. It feels good to talk to people who actually understand me. They are just such incredible people, they are here fighting their own demons, yet they took an hour of their evening to chill with me and help me feel better. On that positive note, I will say goodnight

WEEK 4, DAY 21-27

20.5.19

Weigh day today and I gained which is good. I can't believe its day 21! Lately I've been feeling drained and trapped, locked and institutionalised. I feel suffocated and that I need to see the real world and move my body again. I'm stiff, I can't move, my joints and muscles ache from being in the same position. I'm treated like a number. We all are. I'm either called Room 10 or EA. Some staff don't even remember what my actual name is. I miss being alive. Since being here it feels like my soul has been sucked out of me and been replaced with a battery. This pain is getting too much. My day just hasn't been great either, so my goal is just to hang on and hold on for tomorrow.

We also had an extra community meeting this afternoon which was amazing and so reassuring to know that the other patients feel exactly how I feel. This meeting was for us patients to complain/discuss issues about the unit.

Beep. Beep. Screams…

The fire alarm just went off. A patient has just arrived really distressed and smashed the alarm. I am stressed, I hate loud noises, I hate this. But A and G were so kind and comforted me, and C even gave me her ear defenders. I'm so grateful for the friends I have made here.

The ward felt so unsafe that most of us patients went to the bedroom corridor and cuddled up for a midnight chat. Staff kindly understand that with what was going on we would not be able to sleep at all. It was a hard night; Z was crying and all I could do was try and comfort her. it was hard, but eventually things settled, we gave each other goodnight hugs, laid our heads on our pillows, and got rest so we had energy for the next day.

21.5.19

Ward round and meeting with the solicitor today, hoping they both go well.

Good news finally! In ward round we discussed what leave I should get and it has been decided that I get 2 hours local leave! Yay I am so happy about this; I feel so proud. I get to venture into the outside world, it'll be an adventure!

The solicitor came but no news about the date of my tribunal. Next time I see her we will be looking at notes and statements to make our case.

Bloody awful mood I am in absolute tears. P came to me to tell me that mum can't come every day which I really don't understand because she's my mum and I should not need to have someone control how often I see her. I was starting to get really agitated so P took me for a 10-minute walk to calm me down and talk things through – she is wonderful. Then after the walk I had my psychotherapy which was also relaxing as I got to dance and let out my feelings through movement.

'It's ok to break down, but don't let it win. Don't lie at the bottom forever, rise up and walk again. Feel what you need to feel, but don't let it control you. Give yourself permission to heal and cry, you're doing the best you can'.

22.5.19

It has been a good normal day today. After lunch before going back to school me and staff F (also one of my favourites), played a great game of scrabble. We also had a group today. The groups we have here are Problem Solving, Creative Expression, and Emotional Regulation. These are once weekly from 4.15-5.15, although by 5.10 we are all eager to get out because that is the time that we are allowed my phone. Out of the therapy room and straight to the nurse's office door, queueing for our phones. Oh, the joys of the psych ward.

After dinner I had a 10-minute walk with P, and then a 20-minute walk with granny which was really nice. Then we played scrabble.

It's nearly bed time and I feel really low. I want to leave and have strong urges to harm myself. Anyway, goodnight

23.5.19

I can't believe it's been a month since my birthday. The past week on the ward has been so unsettled and I've felt so bad and gone downhill mood-wise. I got weighed today and put on a bit of weight. I'm so tired of being here, I don't even need to be inpatient anymore. I relapsed yesterday evening, my emotions were just too high and so strong. I've been clean for 5 months...just need to start again. That's the beauty of life, you can always try again. Fall down seven times, stand up eight.

This ward is so toxic. I don't feel safe. There are alarms and banging and yelling. School is becoming such a great escape.

It is getting even more unsettled here, so me, G, C, and student nurse G are playing a card game to distract ourselves. Then thankfully mum came and we went outside for a lovely walk. Goodnight

24.5.19

Even more incidents today. I've been debating whether or not to writ this, but this is my real account of what is happening, so I think its right to mention it. a new boy has come, who I suspect is still high on drugs, and he came too near me, uncomfortably near me, and was about to punch me as well. Luckily, he is being transferred to a more secure hospital. This is meant to be a place of safety but I'd be lying if I said I felt safe right now. One of yesterday's incidents involved 4 police. The staff are so busy with all the incidents that the few of us who aren't having them, are being left out and aren't getting a lot of support as they have no time for us. Anyway, a hug from nurse E gave me a bit of strength.

School has been really enjoyable today, especially the treasure hunt outside. It was nice to roam freely in the garden, and work with each other to find clues. Even better, my team won.

Patient M has had quite a few incidents recently and she looks so battered and worn down, it's so sad to see. Her eyes are bulging and so bruised.

Yay! Ok, this is incredible news. Unexpected, but absolutely wonderful news. Me, my consultant and mum had a meeting together. I screamed and shouted... but...my persuasion worked! Every night I get to go home to sleep as we discussed how it's really affecting my ASD, as the incidents are mainly at night and I feel really unsettled. I am so excited to sleep in my own bed. I can't even express how I feel. Goodnight, I will definitely sleep well tonight.

I really wish I could say that mental health hospitals aren't full of screams that tear your heart and hit your soul. Shouting, alarms, police, restraints, crying and sadness. But, whilst there is all of this pain, things that nobody should ever have to see or hear or live through, there are some of the most wonderful and kind people you will ever come across in these hospitals. There are people who will write little notes and slip them into your diary when you're having a difficult day. You are given hugs, real hugs that make you feel safe. The hugs that touch your heart, that really mean something. You'll meet people who struggle deeply, but is always there to help someone else who is distressed. There are people who will tell you how beautiful you are every single day and how things will get better, when they don't believe it for themselves. These people have lost all hope for themselves but bring so much hope to the people around them. Some people will be so depressed that they hurt themselves and walk around with black, heavy bags under their eyes, and shoulders so low that you can nearly see the weight of the world on them, but will hold your hand for hours, giving you hundreds of reasons not to hurt yourself. Please know this. The person will anxiety is often the best person to know what to say to calm someone down. The person with anorexia will always make you feel gorgeous. The person with PTSD will have big dreams. The person with depression will make you feel worthy of life. These people have severe mental health illnesses, but they are the most amazing people I have ever met. They are absolutely incredible. Struggling, but incredible.

However, this is also the truth of the psych ward:

People in mental health units are at the lowest point in their lives. They need love, care and help. They need treatment. However, many are rejected and failed. You have managers telling patients that if they were so desperate to kill themselves then they'd already have done it. You have nurses calling you liars. Verbally aggressive. Your personal diaries get read and you get searched unnecessarily. Staff will forget to give you your medication and write down that you refused to take it. Staff fall asleep on obs. They may even forget to do the obs. Patients get their hopes up but then they come crashing own because they haven't been accepted for funding. This funding could take them to a place that could actually help them. The use of being threatened to be sectioned is overused and should not be used to scare such vulnerable patients. The mental health act is abused. This is not about every single person who works in these places, there are some incredible staff. But there are people who shouldn't be allowed to work there. I have seen it with my own eyes. And lived the reality. The system is destroyed. People need a healing environment. This really needs sorting out.

25.5.19

So nice to wake up in my own bed. I'm not going to lie, but walking into my home yesterday was very odd and felt weird, and uncomfortable, and new. But I've got used to it again. I am allowed to have breakfast at home, and need to be back at the unit by 8.30. my hard work has paid off and this is such an indescribable feeling. It's so good to know that at the end of each day I know that I will go home to peace and safety, so no matter how terrible the day is, I have something to look forward to in the evening. It was such a shock yesterday; this was not planned whatsoever. In ward round we even talked about how I'm still quite a few weeks off home leave, let alone overnight leave. I just felt like asking again, it doesn't hurt to ask, and this time she said yes. This is one big step forward, and I'm not planning on going back.

Its Saturday but I don't feel as bored because my mood is so good. Mum came after lunch and we drove to a local park for a lovely walk and sat in the sun. I even got a spontaneous ice cream! Recovery win!! It was so nice, relaxing and normal. Then back to the unit for the rest of the afternoon. We did one and a half hours of Hama beads which was a lot of fun and kept us safe and occupied. Then dinner, and then my favourite time of day, home time.

26.5.19

Happy Sunday! Breakfast at homme and then back to the unit. Colouring, and more colouring. I think I have done more colouring here than I've done in the past five years of my life. Then after lunch I went on leave to a local shopping centre and also got a small walk in. Otherwise it has been a normal, good day. Things are looking up.

WEEK 5 DAY 28-34

27.5.19

Morning hair wash. Oh, how good it felt to shower at home, a shower that changes temperature, water that actually goes on your body. Nobody peeking in. just a nice, proper shower. What a luxury!

Back to the unit. I feel a bit self-conscious at the moment. Well, not a bit...very. I've lost all of my muscle and it's just not making me feel great at all. I just feel sluggish and soft and weak. I don't want to lose weight, that business is long gone, but I want to get more muscle which anyway will mean that I put on some weight.

Anyway, mum came and we walked in the park again which was nice. Then more hours of Hama beads and watching the boys do some boxing. Then dinner, then home. Goodnight

28.5.19

Once I got back to the unit I was weighed. I have gained a bit but not as much as I thought. Its half term this week, and also ward round. My psychotherapy was so much fun we danced. Then we had a cooking group as it is half term. I helped make tomato spinach cheese ricotta cannelloni, which I will be having for lunch, and the other option is burgers. Ward round was also good, I still get night leave, and local leave has gone up to 4 hours. Progress! Lunch was so good I enjoyed it. we also had problem solving group, and P bought me two stress balls. At home I went on my first walk in a month. It was so nice, but weird, to be back in familiar fields and parks. I had a bit of a cry before dessert, but fought the voices and listened to extreme hunger.

29.5.19

Back at the unit, and we are making bead bracelets which was fun. Then we did tie dye t-shirts and socks which was so much fun too. It has been such a good busy morning. I'm so glad I went home last night as apparently it was a really awful night here. I've experienced some pretty rough nights here, so I can't even begin to imagine what it would have been like. We had a long community meeting as well, discussing more serious issues. I think this was a follow up from the incidents over the last few days, and the very clear 'domino effect'. Yay there is a unit trip to the cinema to see Aladdin which is so exciting. We were worried it would be cancelled due to the events that have happened, but luckily, they made it happen because today the unit was safe and they felt it was wrong to punish us if we haven't had incidents. It was so good, we went in a taxi, I got a large salted popcorn and Pepsi max, and we watched the movie. Such a great afternoon, and great day in fact. Best day in a very long time.

30.5.19

Day 31! I got weighed, and as expected it has gone up. Then we spent an hour outside painting, so relaxing and fun, and later on emotional regulation, and more bracelet making. Really fun and busy day.

31.5.19

Morning. I can't wait for tomorrow as it is Saturday and I have 4 hours leave., I'm so excited. The staff and patient are so proud of me of getting to where I am, and it's so lovely to hear all their positive comments. I had a nice catch up with P who is so happy about my progress, and shocked at how well I'm doing. Then we all had an at group which was good. At home I had one of the loveliest walks yet, and was able to sit on a hill, watching the sun set with mum, it was magical and so special. My soul really felt at peace, and I was in awe of the natural beauty of this world.

1.6.19

I'm so happy that I'm only at the unit for 4 and a half hours today. On the weekend I only need to be here at 10, and I have 4 hours local leave. My overnight leave starts at6 so 6-4 is 2. Therefore, I can be here at 10 and then leave just after 2, this is great I am loving this, 4 hours is nothing. I am in such a good place right now. Best afternoon, I went to Primark, and really treated myself with retail therapy. Then I got a large smoothie with all the extras!! Who is this girl? Granny also came home to see me and we played some uno. Long gone are the days spent with no leave, being on obs and being watched like a naughty toddler. I have earned my freedom and will continue earning it. I am on my way to discharge.

2.6.19

Happy Sunday! Went to unit, stayed 4 hours, then ventured into the world. What more can I say?

WEEK FIVE DAY 35-41

3.6.19

So, I know things have been good lately and I am getting more leave, but I do still feel rubbish, and cry and get angry. Now the staff think I'm doing bad and don't want to send me home which is ridiculous. This place is awful. I didn't even gain a lot of weight. One of my good friends J is getting discharged today, I will really miss her. We've become early morning buddies, school buddies, and she gives such good hugs. I am really going to miss her. She is like my little sister. We had her leaving tea which was amazing, and I had her cake!! Then group. Luckily the issues form this morning got sorted out and I could go home like usual.

4.6.19

Ward round today. I hope it goes well; I have been continuing with the progress.

Bad. Ward. Round.

Absolutely no positives were said, I have no leave and no exercise. I asked questions like why, and they got angry at me and wouldn't respond. I have done so much and tried so hard and it feels like I am getting punished. I am getting punished. I was so sad so therapist K sat with me outside for a while which was really nice. I thought ward round would go well. They didn't even ask how I was or any god things, it was straight into the negatives and it stayed that way. I am so sad and angry right nw. at least I have the support of my friends here; they are my rocks.

For the first time I was allowed to do yoga at school which was the most calming thing ever, the lights were dim, there was bergamot incense, and the teacher was amazing.

For some reason now I'm allowed home? I am confused. Life right now is one big question mark.

'*We will be okay. We will grow. We will flourish. We will be happy. The storm we're going through right now is there to clear our path. It feels like we are swimming endlessly and there's no shore in sight, but keep swimming. Keep swimming even when you're sure you'd rather drown. You're swimming because your enemies can't swim. Keep fighting even when it's scary. One day you will be happy, and you'll wake up and run downstairs for breakfast and laugh and smile, with no enemy to run away from anymore*'

5.6.19

Hoping for a better day and maybe some answers. It has been a day. Just a day. I can't tell if it has been good, bad, normal, or any adjective to be honest. It has just been a day. Mum bought me a lovely suitcase, so that was one good thing and it's also reminding me how much I need to get out before July when I go on holiday. Otherwise, today has just been a day.

6.5.19

I did some yoga outside for ten minutes – perks of being at home – I can wake up whenever and do some calming things in my own time, outside when the sun is rising, birds chirping...bliss, in contrast to either someone screaming or staff waking you up, going to the same dark lounge.

Back at the unit, I got weighed and have gained. In school there was pe but as usual I can't do it. since it is a warm day I wanted to sit outside for a bit, but five minutes later we had to go in because the unit was short staffed. So annoying. We had emotional regulation today. I enjoy the groups, they're fun, good therapists and it takes up time.

Then mum came as a huge surprise after the group to take me for a short shopping trip, and got back in time for dinner. That was a really nice surprise. And then got to go home again.

7.6.19

So, great (not) start to the morning. I came to the unit and was left in the entrance for 40 minutes as I was forgotten to be collected. I feel really important...

Anyway, I met with a social worker today, she seems nice. I also had art therapy which was good, and played a bit of football with the patients. I'm not allowed to walk especially long walks but I am allowed to do some light sports which is nice so I can join in and move around a tiny bit. I've got my full leave back now, so I can go home for dinner which I am pleased about. Home dinners are so much better than the hospital food which I struggle to even call a meal. Goodnight

8.6.19

Back to the unit for my short Saturday stay. A staff here remembers me from my first admission and just told me – 'do you remember me, you weren't very happy then', and that has made me realise how far I have come. That sentence really hit hard.

Time has whizzed by and dad is about to come. We are going to a nearby lovely town for a walk, shops, and snack at a milkshake bar. It was a lovely Saturday afternoon, and it felt so good to just be able to go home straight after.

9.6.19

Day 41! I can't believe how many days it has been. At the unit I'm currently just sitting outside in the sun, it is so warm. I also did some gardening with G and staff J which was so fun and nice to do something physical but calm. That pretty much took up the day, and after lunch I got picked up by mum ad dad. We went to get a smoothie, and then went to the cinema...and even after my big smoothie I got some pick'n'mix. I've had such a nice normal weekend, and I feel so happy and pleased. Goodnight

WEEK 6 DAY 42-48

10.6.19

Weigh day, and I gained as expected. I saw an educational psychologist (who knew they existed?) today which was interesting. He is supposed to help in some way or another with getting back into school since I haven't been in education for one and a half years, until coming to the hospital school. I guess a suitable school needs to be found for me.

11.6.19

CPA today...hoping for even more leave. I feel quite bad today, and I'm very nervous for the CPA. The weather is bad, it's just one of those days where I can't wait for it to end. I had my psychotherapy today which was so pleasing to the soul, I pretty much just slammed a yoga ball into the floor and let it bounce to the ceiling repetitively. After lunch before school I played a game of scrabble with staff D, and K and G. then in school we had pig pong which I was allowed to do although I am awful at it.

CPA was not good. I am frustrated, no news things are just staying the same. Afterwards I was really upset so P stayed with me for half an hour, she is amazing. She was with me in the CPA and we wrote to each other on paper.

Later on, I went home, and cried and shouted. My emotions had to be let out and released. The evening was super challenging and I almost had to return to the unit, but luckily, I just about managed to pull myself together and calm down. Goodnight

12.6.19

I'm not going to the unit this morning as I have some appointments that I have been allowed to go to. I had to go to the opticians, and then went to Home Sense (the book section is my favourite). Then I had an appointment with my surgeon – I had otoplasty a few weeks before I got admitted, so this was a vital post op check-up.

I got back to the unit for lunch, and then did some art at school. It was actually really nice not to go to the unit this morning. Group today was really fun, we paired up, asked each other questions completely unrelated to our illnesses, and shared it with the rest of the groups.

It was another slightly hard evening at home but I got through it. Goodnight

13.6.19

I'm scared I will get in trouble if the staff don't think I can manage at home because it's been tough the past few nights. Oh sh*t I haven't gained weight, I hope they don't punish me. This day has really not gotten off to the best start.

Omg. So even though I didn't gain, for the first time ever I was allowed to go to the gym to do pe!! Yay!!!! I did 10 minutes on the bike, 5 minutes rowing, and 20 minutes badminton. It felt amazing to move my body, and it was so lovely to go into an actual leisure centre with normal people and just forget about the situation.

I saw my doctor and she reassured me that I haven't lost my leave or got punished which is good, and she said I am possibly getting discharged in 3 weeks. This afternoon has been incredible. However, she also said that I could be getting discharged onto a CTO, which lasts for 6 months. It means that I am still under the mental health act and have a list of community rules to adhere to. These include going to school, appointments, eating and not being aggressive. If I break a rule, I am automatically recalled for a 72-hour admission.

Then I had emotional regulation, and straight after that I went home. Goodnight

14.6.19

Breakfast. Unit. School. Snacks and meals ...the usual. Had a small game of scrabble with K, and then had art therapy. It's A's last therapy and I am going to miss her so much. She was one of my first friends, and we have become close. She always plaits my hair, and she is my lunch buddy. I will be so sad to see her go but I am extremely proud of her. Her leaving tea was so emotional and full of tears. She even gave me a hug telling me that shed miss being lunch buddies with me, and gave me a card. I will never ever forget her.

I went home and had a good evening.

15.9.19

Patient L is pregnant at 17 which is really sad. She has shown me a side to life I haven't experienced. Her mum was unfortunately a heroin addict whilst pregnant with her, and so L now has really damaged joints, especially her shoulder which dislocates often. I hope life works out for L, she is a lovely girl and deserves the best opportunities, and I hope she begins to realise that.

As its Saturday I left early again an went to the lovely old town, where we found a cute café where I had the most delicious home-made peanut butter vegan cup which was huge, and a smoothie with blueberries, strawberries, raspberries, maca, coconut water and maple syrup. So yummy. Then quickly to the shops and then home. Great day

16.6.19

It's Sunday! I am at home all day today. Yes, you read that right, home all day. For the first time in 48 days am spending the whole day and night at home. I am so proud of myself as I have worked so hard to get to this point. To celebrate, mum and dad took me to London, where we stumbled upon a really cool prison museum. Then we walked along the Thames and stopped for my first real restaurant meal in over a year, in Wagamama. I can't even explain how it felt to be free I London, living normally, and having an actual meal.

Today has been the best day yet, and my heart is bursting with happiness.

WEEK 7 DAY 49-55

School was great today. From 10-10.45 we prepped for the BBQ, so we got the garden sorted with chairs, rugs, bunting and tables. Then quick snack break, and then a bit more prepping. From 12.30-2 we all just chilled in the garden having a BBQ, this was amazing. We had food that we'd made, rugs and mats, music, all in the sun, surrounded with laughter, and staff popping in from the unit across the road. This was so lovely I cannot even describe it. Then at the unit we had 15 minutes of mindfulness laying in the unit's patio outside which was so relaxing, and I had a 10 minutes session with P. this day could not be any better. Then we had problem solving group, and then garden games in the patio such as tennis.

By the time I knew it, mum was here to pick me up. Sunny days in recovery, surrounded by love and joy are moments that will stay with me forever.

18.6.19

Really fun session with D in psychotherapy, and then ward round. Nothing new, I still need to gain weight and have the same amount of leave. No negative comments whatsoever for the first time so that's great. Yoga at school was amazing! Then home. Goodnight, I'm feeling good.

19.6.19

I met with a tribunal doctor today. Other than that, a normal routine, however I am feeling a bit sick today sweating really badly with headaches. Night, don't have much energy to write today

20.6.19

Staff F said she loves my height and said I'd look epic in heels...I love the relationship I have got with the people to work here. I was allowed in the gym again today which was great, I did 10 minutes on the bike, 20 minutes badminton, 10 minutes football. It has been a good busy day. I met with my solicitor for one and a half hours, going through papers and things about the tribunal. Then home.

21.6.19

I've just had a normal morning at the unit. But, I've been allowed to leave today during lunch, to go and see my old friends from my old school, it was so nice, I went to the school, and since one of them lives on the same road, we went to her house, and had the best catchup and ate lunch. It was so amazing I loved it and I'm so happy we were able to do it.

I had the tribunal today, and it went wrong. It was awful I don't even want to write about it. Bad mood, goodnight

22-23.6.19

I am at home all weekend. Its day 54! Today I'm just relaxing in the garden, and going to a beauty salon to get my brows and lashes tinted. I'm not a girly girl, but the feminine things that I like to do regularly are getting my brows and lashes done, and painting my nails. I also went on a lovely walk, and have just been eating loads. What more could I ask for?

It is Sunday and I'm sad because last night was hard. I'm just crying now in the garden with mum. Thankfully granny came to save the day and took me for a nice walk and out for lunch. It has been a very confusing day today, so I'll leave it at this. Goodnight

WEEK 8 DAY 56-62

24.6.19

Back at the unit. We had a school trip to a museum which was really fun, and had a tiny walk in the surrounding park. Apparently, I am very close to being weight restored!! Problem solving group, then home. I knew weight gain would happen, but it was hard. Painful even, not just mentally, but physically. My blood pressure and pulse would go all over the place, my blood sugar levels were crazy, my face puffed up like a chipmunk, and my stomach was in agony. It would bloat more than I'd ever thought was possible. But the thing about gaining weight and reaching a point where you are healthy, is that you will probably hate it. You might feel huge and uncomfortable, and feel as if you are in somebody else's body. And that's okay, but don't forget that this is where your body will be happy and your bones will be strong. Eventually you will accept it, and over time you will love it. Nobody told me about the physical pain of gaining weight, and that's all whilst dealing with the mental struggles. I watched my body grow. My thighs stopped touching each other, I could no longer count every single one of my ribs, my jawline to longer stuck out, nor did the bones on my hands. However, the hair that was falling out soon started to strengthen, my nails grew again, my eyes weren't sunken anymore, but full of life. I didn't exhaust myself walking 5 metres, I didn't see a galaxy of stars when I stood up and living no longer seemed pointless. My clothes became tighter, but that's ok, they look better on me now, and I can buy myself loads of new clothes. I was becoming alive again. Beautifully alive. My meal plan was also hard, I'll tell you that. It felt like I was always eating and my portions were huge... but guess what, nothing lasts forever.

25.6.19

Today is just another normal day. Ward round was good, nothing has changed, and dance therapy was good. I'm really running out of things to write about now, which I guess isn't a bad thing at all.

26.6.19

We had a school trip to an animal museum today which was cool. I actually fell asleep in the minivan according to G. I'm enjoying this week of school trips and the sun.

27.6.19

Gym today! Machines for 40 minutes was good. Sat in the unit patio for a bit this lunch which was good. They also forgot my snack today...I got away with it.

28.6.19

We had a school trip, my favourite of the week, to an aircraft museum, and P came with and went around with me and even bought me a snack. Then we also stopped off at the RSPCA, but me and P didn't want to go in, so instead we sat on the grass and played cards together until the others came back. I had the best time with her and the trip was so good. So good.

Very big news... as of today I am discharged onto a CTO, I cannot believe it. I'm still coming in next week, but I am extremely proud and happy I am so shocked. I can't believe I'm actually writing this when 60 days ago I was writing the complete opposite.

I am so happy to be discharged, but I also have this sad pit in my stomach. I've become family with the people here, and I will so deeply miss them, especially P. I've gotten used to waking up to lots of good mornings. I've gotten used to the routine and the people. I will miss school and groups and therapy and the good days, but I definitely won't miss the bad days.

29-30.6.19

Happy weekend. Just hanging about and enjoying life, not much more to say.

WEEK 9 day 63-65

1.7.19

I saw P today and we walked around the hospital grounds and sat on a bench for a chat. Apparently patient M had told her something good about me but she wasn't allowed to share what it was. I was with P for ages it was so nice. I love K, she asked me to write her a letter so she can remember me. M is leaving today, I like her a lot, and she has come so far. We had her leaving tea and I had some of her cake! Granny picked me up today and I just had a normal evening.

2.7.19

I had my last psychotherapy today which was so emotional, and also my last ward round. I am still in shock. I'm really upset about saying bye to my psychotherapist, she has honestly helped me so much and it's always been a highlight of my week. She has this vibe about her that I can really connect to, which is rare as I find it difficult to connect to therapists usually, so now that I finally have her and P it makes me sad to leave them. It was my last yoga today too. It's a day full of lasts, but opening up to a life full of firsts and beginnings.

3.7.19

So, this is it, I guess. My heart and mind are all over the place, I feel happy, scared and so sad. I have made it through the first stage of recovery. I have grown so much, not just in size, but in happiness. This has been such a difficult journey with tears and anger, pain and frustration, and endless amounts of guilt. But it has also been so beautiful to watch myself come back to me. My journey to happiness is beginning now, and I am so ready to make my life better, and become stronger. It's so hard to even think about how much I've changed in the past two months and it's scary but so beautiful.

I had a meeting where I cried so hard to P, and then she came with me to sign the wall. That was a special moment. 6 times a day in the dining room I have looked at that wall, scanning everyone's names, finding a place to write mine, wondering if that day would ever come. For P to be with me, was special, and it felt so emotional to finally write my name on it. I gave my last goodbyes and hugs. I can't deal with this feeling.

This has been a tough but magical journey to being alive again. I have so far to go, but this is a huge step forward. No matter how hard things have been and will be, I am moving on. I'm looking at my old life now one more time, and I will take a deep breath and whisper, 'I will never see you again'.

Am I brave yet?

My ocean of thoughts and words

A lot of us are happy but sad. Surrounded by people yet so alone. We love ourselves but hate ourselves. We're proud but guilty. We're hopeful but hopeless. We see the light, we do. But we can't tell if it's the sun or the fire. And that is what makes us scared to go on, because it could be the light we've been looking for, but it could also be the fire that burns.

Writing this has resurfaced some painful memories. I wish I could grab the vulnerable and broken me at the beginning and show her how far she will go, and that everything will be okay. It's amazing to see how at the beginning I wrote about pain and not being able to get through it, and at the end I transformed into someone with hope and a future. I want to show you that it is possible to make it, that no matter how deep inside the rut you are, you can still get out and start living again.

My mind is a kingdom. There are dangerous cities and beautiful mountains. There are deep, dark woods and beautiful flower gardens. There are monsters and there are angels. Sometimes I get lost in the city of pain and fear. Sometimes the monsters capture me. Sometimes I get trapped in the terrifying woods and think there's no way out. Sometimes I feel free at the top of the mountains. Sometimes I'm happy amongst the pretty flowers. Sometimes I'm at peace because the angels are there. My mind is a kingdom, a kingdom only I know. I can get so lost in it that I forget I'm human. My kingdom is my escape. I either escape to a place of hope or fall into the traps that possess me.

Strength doesn't come from winning. Strength is going through tough times, choosing not to surrender. Your struggles develop your strengths. It's in our darkest moments that we must remember the light. So, from now on I am going to ask myself what makes me come alive. And that's what I will do, because I've been lost in the dark for too long. This world needs more people who have become alive, and I will do that. I am going to turn this pain into something beautiful. I've been dead for too long and now I'm starting to live; I have a feeling it's going to be wonderful.

This is a complete change of subject, but I want to write it now, and be real with you, showing the reality of writing this book. I am writing this with so much doubt. What if it's not good? What if I'm over sharing? Or under sharing? What if it doesn't work out? What will people think? Don't let doubt feed your soul and mind, making you believe you cannot do something. This is my story and my experience and my best tips to help you, and I think I'm starting to realise there is no wrong way to write this. I hope you understand that the diary entries were pretty much typed word for word, and is not meant to be like a story whatsoever. If I were to change and edit a lot, it would take way the realness, and I want you to read the exact words I wrote in the worst of times. After everything that I've gone through and seen, I can't keep quiet and let this kind of suffering continue. This book may make you feel uncomfortable, and in the kindest way possible, that is exactly how I want you to feel. If you feel comfortable reading this, then I haven't achieved my goal. I want you to feel uncomfortable because that feeling is what will help break the stigma. That feeling will educate you. Mental illness is not meant to be comfortable, nothing about being sick is comfortable, and it's not supposed to be easy to talk about. But we can't continue to shy away from the truth and sugar coat reality. I hope that although some parts are upsetting to read, you feel hopeful and have a better understanding of some of the issues that I have written about.

Institutionalisation is hard. There are rigid routines and fears of the outside world. A song can cause memories flooding back to me from a song that we often listened to over and over again. Screams and shouts and alarms can hurt and pierce my soul. It's hard having to get used to taking your own medication, eating and keeping safe. It can be so hard to get used to it but please know that it will work out. You will adjust and get through it and live a happy life free from the walls of a hospital. Because being inpatient isn't a holiday camp. Not at all. You don't sign up to go there to make best friends and relax. Inpatient isn't something that happens to everyone, it's the last option when all others have been tried and exhausted. There is absolutely nothing beautiful or 'cool' about it. Imagine being pinned down to the floor with five people on top of you, pulling your trousers down to inject you. Imagine if you've been raped and this pushes you off the edge, bringing back memories of that trauma.

Imagine showering with staff watching you. Imagine sleeping with someone watching you. Inpatient is hearing the alarm go off and fearing the worst. It's watching and hearing someone you were talking to five minutes ago hurt themselves. It's being sat at a table, forced to eat, with most people having their heads down and crying, struggling to even pick up the fork. You face your worst fears when you're inpatient. There is no option to escape. Once you're in, the only way out is through.

And I know I've made a lot of progress, but it still hurts to look back. Looking at pictures, eating certain foods, even going to certain places is hard. I still have nightmares and flashbacks, I still cry strong, burning tears when I think about the old me. It feels as if I can actually touch my suffering…feel how much it hurt, how scary it was. I can transport myself back in time to those miserable days, and I know for sure that I don't ever want to live like that again. I think I miss being sick sometimes, but deep down I know that I don't. What I actually miss is the feeling of control. The euphoria of restriction and the galaxy that greeted me whenever I stood up. I don't miss my eating disorder though, not at all. I realise now that I have been brainwashed into thinking that an illness is the only thing that makes me special. Missing anorexia was always going to happen. You see, that was how I coped for so long. That was who I became, I didn't know anything else. I had nothing else. It took up 24 hours of my day, stealing my identity. I lost my hobbies and friends and enjoyments. And there is something so strangely comforting about being ill. Maybe you want to look like you did when you weren't doing too well. Maybe you felt comforted having people worry about you. Maybe you miss your addictions because of the feeling they gave you. Starving doesn't make you special, it makes you sick. It is called an illness for a reason, it's not healthy and it huts you and those around you. That comfort is fake, because comfort shouldn't damage you. I feel afraid to give up that identity, because my true self has been hijacked by the demons and replaced with an illness. I know that I will never become 'her' again. I have to move on and become me, and for that, I am grieving the old me, so I can let the present me grow without being held down by the heavy chains, so that I can properly say goodbye to her and live a new beautiful life. I must not mourn for the body I once had because it was completely broken and unloved and uncared for. I need to focus on loving and healing my body, and also loving the person who lives inside it. when I look in the mirror, I need to understand that I don't need to cry for the girl I no longer see, she is gone. I will celebrate who I am, she is beautiful and free.

I am grieving over a girl who died. She had dark eyes, broken lips, cracked nails and split hair. Her body was a cage, her mind was a battlefield. One day she died, it was scary and painful, it was lonely and unsafe. But life gave her another chance. She had bright eyes and rosy red lips, beautiful nails and golden hair. Her body was her home and her mind was a galaxy with the brightest stars. I'm grieving over a girl, that girl was me. But I am celebrating new life, the life I'm creating.

In the depths of my disorder I didn't want help and said nothing was wrong. I was focused on destroying myself, and saw nothing wrong with that. I was empty and hollow, with no self-appreciation. And like I've already said, I miss having the ability to feel nothing. No emotions, no pain. Absolutely nothing. But then there comes a point where you can only take so much, and it's time to find peace, which is exactly what I'm doing. I'm a work in progress.

For quite a while I have found that mental health has turned into a competition. You can't discuss depression because they've attempted suicide 5 times and you haven't tried at all. You can't talk about self-harm because they have stitches and you only have a mark. Every single time you want to reach out you don't because you don't think you're sick enough. You would not have that attitude with cancer. If you have cancer then you get treatment. So why is it that with mental health illnesses you have to tick boxes and wait until you're dying to receive appropriate care. I've also found that this 'how sick are you' stigma has come from the NHS. I was only taken seriously for my mental health illnesses once they got to quite a critical stage. I reached out for help at beginning like everyone says you should do, but there was no one on the other side to help me when it was the early stages of the illness. When I went to a&e one of the first times, I was in early stages of anorexia. The doctor asked to weigh me and do a test, can I squat and stand up. Because my weight wasn't dramatically low and I was still eating relatively decently and I succeeded in the squat test, I was told that I couldn't be diagnosed with an eating disorder. A few months later I was in a critical condition in that same a&e, and was then told I had anorexia. By that point my mind has been completely taken over and I was deep into the illness. My suicide attempts have never been dramatic. I've felt like such a fake and burden going into hospital; just another teenager who wanted to find a way out. I felt like a waste of time and it felt like I was wasting the money of the NHS. And unfortunately, this is how it is for so many people, and from the moment we reach out we have the idea of not being sick enough drilled into our minds.

I asked 129 people from the ages of 14-25 to vote for whether mental health care in both the community and hospitals has shocked them, and these were the results – 84% yes 16% no. I find these numbers terrible, and it should be the other way round.

I also asked them if they've been inpatient before, and if they had, did they find it a toxic environment. The results were 75% yes 25% no, also absolutely shocking figures. An inpatient environment should be healing and safe, yet three quarters of young people found it toxic. 'Some things I saw were quite traumatic and I felt like I came out with more problems than when I went in' – anonymous

I want mental health to be so normalised that young children can tell their parents how they are feeling, if they're feeling mentally ill, just like they would if they had a stomach ache or painful tooth. I want mental health to be so normalised that school lets you go home after a panic attack or depressive episode just like they would if you sustain an injury. I want mental health to be so normalised that when someone is in recovery, the people around them care and nurture them, asking for progress reports and sending get well soon cards, just like they would for any other sort of recovery. I want mental health to be normalised because every single mental disorder is just as scary and damaging as a life threatening injury, and unfortunately we live in a society where we pass people by everyday who are so unwell in this sense but don't receive even a fraction of the care they deserve just because their illness is unseen.

I hope I live to see the day in which mental health is normalised, and the funding improves. I hope I live to see the day in which self-harm scars aren't stated at and demonised. I hope I live to see the day in which, regardless of weight or size or race, those with eating disorders are treated equally and not denied treatment just because of a weight criteria. I hope I live to see the day in which the suicide rate decreases. I hope I live in a day where cellulite and stretch marks are normal and no person advertises for anti-cellulite cream. I hope I live in a world where fat phobia doesn't exist anymore and being gay is seen as normal. I hope I live to see every human being treating themselves with respect and kindness.

This generation is too broken. We're dead but still walking, hidden and beautifully lost. We are the generation of pills that are supposed to make us feel, accidental overdoses and overprescribed meds. In this generation people drown themselves in alcohol alone, or injecting drugs into our veins to try and make the sadness go away. The generation of needles, pills and shot glasses. We're the generation where we need to be academically competitive, panic attacks, hollow eyes and perfect marks. We are the generation of skipped dances and skipped meals, self-loathing and heartbreak. We are the generation...the generation of the future. So, to the future generation, I hope you fall in love with being alive and see it as a blessing. I hope you learn to understand that life is so much more than getting a snapchat from a boy you won't even remember in two years' time. I hope you have friends that give you joy, and I even hope that you get in trouble together. I hope you'll make memories for life, laughing and screaming at the top of your lungs, free, taking too many pictures. I hope you know that you can do anything, but it will take hard work. Please don't just sit around complaining about the things that you wish could change, because I hope you are the change. I hope you treat yourself just as well as you treat the people around you. I hope you fall in love with being alive.

A big, very big issue, is underfunding. I'm not usually the politics type of girl, but there's a few things I'd like to mention. Mental health services are getting far less support than physical hospitals and services. Think about this, there was one day where the unit was extremely short staffed, and pretty much most were bank nurses who didn't know us. Now, they are the loveliest people, kind and caring, but that doesn't mean they are able to do certain jobs. On the meal plan table, a girl who was in a bad place, got given a large meal. Her supporter told her 'even I couldn't eat that much, leave some if you want'. Even writing this infuriates me. She was a severely underweight teenager who was on a calorie-controlled meal plan and needed to eat that. No staff, no human being should comment on portion sizes. That poor girl ended up having serious incidents and put on bed rest. If only there was more funding and we could've had workers who knew more about the patients, especially the diagnosis itself and the fact that they have an eating disorder.

For Mental Health Awareness Week 2020 UK, the theme was kindness. The truth is, I am fed up of awareness. Yes, awareness does help to a certain extent, but a lot of it misses the point and leaves many sufferers frustrated. The popular saying of 'just talk' and 'be kind' and 'reach out' means absolutely nothing if a person cannot access the right care. Nothing feels as unkind as feeling suicidal yet being told you're not 'suicidal enough' to get help and support, which is actually happening here in the UK. It has happened to me. So, what would be kind? Mental health services being *funded*. Computer systems that are fast and actually work. Staff that actually get proper training. There should be more investment in access to help and not having to be turned away or put on a ridiculous waiting list, or when you've finally got to your appointment, your therapist has barely been trained and doesn't know what to do with you. instead of people posting images about kindness, let's actually act on it and give people the care they really deserve.

F*ck wearing yellow.

F*ck raising 'awareness'.

F*ck celebrities and politicians encouraging us to talk about our feelings.

I'm sure we are all aware by now. We are talking.

But there are no funds. There are dangerous life-threatening long waiting lists to even get an initial assessment and lack of specialised care. Please fund, that is the biggest act of support and kindness you can do.

We are told to reach out for help, but I'm afraid to say there is nothing to reach out to other than a waiting list a yearlong and people telling you that you're fine. People support mental health until it becomes real. People support depression until they see someone in a scary depressive episode. people support anxiety until they get annoyed that their friend won't see them. People will support eating disorders until they get tired of seeing you say no to an apple, because it's not that bad, is it? it seems as if mental health has become a trend. It's 'cool' to share your story and get publicity. No, it is not cool. It is not a trend. This 'trend' is blinding people into thinking the stigma is going. No, the stigma is growing. 'love Island XYZ said she had depression and started working out and is now the happiest she's ever been, don't pretend to still be sick when it's so easy to be okay.' 'This singer had an eating disorder and is thriving now after getting treatment, what's taking you so long'. Instagram is filled with people posting images saying you are good enough, yet these same people also promote weight loss pills. Mental illness is romanticised. Put #depressed and you will find millions of photos of girls with roses on their wrists, boys with hoodies and quotes saying 'help me, I want to disappear'.

There's also been a flood of social media campaigns encouraging people to speak openly about their mental health. Social media has rushed to express their own genuine emotional distress with the intention of helping to normalize, destigmatize, and relate to those struggles. In our haste, though, we may have forgotten the fundamental and very important distinction between feeling sad and the terms used to diagnose mental disorders, for example anxiety and depression. People label their sadness as depression and their nervousness as anxiety when the problems that they're facing often don't reflect those psychological problems. It's normal to get sad and anxious, they're emotions that we all feel, but it does not mean that they are serious mental illnesses such as depression and anxiety. If healthy people are convinced that they're depressed, they ultimately identify with the glamorized social media posts, pushing the boundaries even more. Social media has blurred this line between what is true mental illness and what is performance. (Some influencers are absolutely wonderful though and save many lives).

"More and more teenagers are convinced that depression, anxiety, anorexia, and bipolarity are 'cool' or can make you 'special,'" says Rola Jadayel, another co-author of the social media study and professor of sciences at the University of Balamand in Lebanon.*"There's this group think that starts to believe that's all mental illness is: some mild anxiety and a breathing exercise,"* she says. *"It normalizes a version of mental illness that isn't realistic for those of us who actually have serious mental illness. Someone with severe anxiety disorder is going to need a whole heck of a lot more than breathing exercises, you know."*

When the outside hurts as much as the inside

If you're thinking about self-harming for the first time, please don't ever start. You may think 'oh it's just this once' but what starts out as a small scratch one time will turn into something worse. It will become a painful and scary habit. It will isolate you. Please don't ever start. You don't have to suffer alone, and there are healthier, safe ways to cope with what you're going through.

Before my eating disorder had begun, I was self-harming, feeling low and anxious. When I first self-harmed, it was just a little flick of a switch, a small shudder. It wasn't anything dramatic like the media made it seem but it was the beginning of an endless dig into a deep hole. It wasn't an addiction yet, and I wasn't far down the ladder I'd have to climb to get out of it, but I stayed in it. It wasn't all scars down my wrists and sunflowers painted on them like Instagram said it would be like. Instead it was friendships crushed and dreams destroyed. And by then, I was too far down the ladder to even believe the top was reachable.

I want to try and help you understand self-harm. YoungMinds say that 1 in 12 young people self-harm, with 10% of 15-16-year olds doing it. People don't really self-harm to die, it's more of a way of dealing with life. It's not really something that you can get to grips with unless you struggle with it. The most important thing I want you to know is that it is not for attention. Do you understand how much self-hatred someone must have to hurt themselves? If self-harm was for attention, we would do it in your face. Not barricade the bathroom doors, cover up with long sleeves no matter how hot it is, do it in places no one would think of looking at, look ashamed when someone sees it, even be ashamed of yourself. So no, self-harm is in no way attention seeking. Not at all. I hope you haven't gotten yourself into the vicious cycle of self-destruction. Because this is what will happen…you will get addicted. It will drive you ridiculously insane. You'll crave it, rush to get home, run to your room and a few minutes later breathe a large sigh of relief. You'll start to find you hate your body even more than before because now it has marks and scars on it. You'll cut for a week, then a month, then a year and so on. I hope you realise you will be sore; a single movement could hurt your skin. You'll try to stop hurting yourself, but the pain of trying will be so much that you *have* to start again. And wait. What happens if you accidentally cut too deep? Or your burn gets infected? You can't tell anyone because no one can know. But at the same time, you know you really need help. Self-harm isn't pretty or healthy, and I really want you to know that it's not worth it. You don't deserve to hurt your beautiful skin. It's illogical yet so logical at the same time, and the urges are like those of alcohol and drugs. And scars…we are not proud of them. I certainly am not. They are not beautiful. They are not what I want to see when I look at myself. My scars show that I crumbled, and tell stories of my sadness. They remind me of the constant darkness and the times I had to be saved. They take me back to the days when I was afraid of living. My scars are marks of an illness. They're not pretty. They itch. They never let me forget that this horrible addiction has made itself a comfortable home in my mind.

If you're a relative of someone who harms themselves, know it's not your fault. Make sure you let the person know you care for them, but don't follow them around like a puppy unless told to by services. You may think about removing sharp objects from the home, and in some cases that's helpful, however in some cases it's not because that is their only way to cope. Be patient. They may not want to talk about it at first, wait for them to be ready. And please remember to look after yourself.

Make a survival plan:

1. When you're in a calm state of mind, think about things that will help you be safe. Boxing? Art? Baking? Ice cubes on your body? Be with your pet. Snap a rubber band on your wrist. Drive. Scream. Write down how you feel and then tear it up.
2. Write these down so when you're struggling you can look at the page and choose something nice to do.

Yes, I have cut myself. Yes, I have scars. But at least I'm still here. I know that I would much rather have permanent scars than the alternative permanent solution, death. Yes, I have hit rock bottom and considered suicide many ties, and starved myself for days. But it is still better than ending my life. So much better. And I am so tired of being told to cover up because people think I'm a freak or dangerous. The truth is, we choose life every single day, and I am proud of myself and every single person out there holding on.

Why do I think I'm stuck in this cycle? Honestly, I don't know. It's addictive in the sickest way possible. There's something about having control that feels so powerful. There is something so relieving and releasing about it. And I really feel like I deserve it. I've been a very toxic person to some people when I was really struggling, and I have done things that I so strongly and deeply regret. I've done things I should never have done, and hurt people. I can't get away with it so easily, I need to hurt myself because I deserve to feel the pain that I've caused to others. As a child at school we'd always be warned of the dangers of sharp objects, and we'd carefully cut out pictures whilst making Mother's Day cards, laughing and fully of happiness. 10 years later and paper has turned into skin. Instead of making cards of love I make lines of hatred. Sometimes I just need to feel something. Something other than numbness or guilt or sadness, and self-harm is my way of coping, which you could argue isn't really a proper way of coping. The scariest thing is the realisation that you are addicted to something. Whether it is alcohol, cigarettes, self-harm or drugs, you know you are addicted when you tell yourself 'this is my last…'. But the thing is you can't just stop, because an addiction is an obsession that takes over your mind and nearly every thought. What I find sad about that is that there was once a time when I didn't understand the idea and concept. I couldn't wrap myself around the 'why'.

Why would someone do this to themselves? Sadly, now, I know. I know that emptiness that fills you, and that desperation for something that will make you feel different. Something that'll turn the hurt into something else. I don't want to self-harm, I don't want to hurt myself. But it's an addiction. A completely illogical and painful addiction, but nevertheless, an addiction. Last cut, I say. And I get through the day. But then the urges come, even on a good day. You see, it started off as a way to feel, to cope, but now it's the feeling. You know you want to, the demons say, and so I hurt, because I feel alive, because I can't stop.

But I won't stop talking about this, and we can't stop helping others until this is a thing of the past.

If the mountain seems too big to climb today, start with zipping up your coat and packing your rucksack. If the ocean seems too large to swim across today, dip your toes in the water and start making friends with the dolphins. If the storm seems too dangerous to walk through this evening, start with writing a plan and rest under a shelter. If life seems too hard today, start with knowing you don't have to climb a mountain or swim a whole ocean today, but still do a small task, anything that will help you move forwards.

PART TWO

The facts

Diet Culture

Diet culture[1] – a set of beliefs that send out an idea that 'thin' bodies are ideal, beautiful, healthy and desirable. It conveys that foods are either 'good' or 'bad', and that you will be more worthy if you have a smaller body or eat 'healthily'. I think we can all agree that in today's society, there is too much diet culture. Far too much.

Eat five small meals per day and run. Also, only way breakfast lunch and dinner and walk. Eat lots of protein and lift weights, it's good for your joints. Also, don't eat protein and do cardio. Don't be sedentary. But don't be too active either. Make sure you replace your lost salt, but don't eat too much sodium. Protein also hurts your kidneys, but make sure you eat a lot of it for good health. Drink water. Don't over hydrate. Don't starve yourself…unless you call it 'intermittent fasting', and then it's okay to starve yourself a little bit, finding something to control. Get some sun every day, don't get cancer.

---

[1] Erica Leon Nutrition. (2016). Erica Leon Nutrition. [online] Available at: https://ericaleon.com/.

I asked 163 people from the ages of 14-25 to answer two questions, here are the results:

Are you usually comfortable and happy with the way you look? – 17% yes 83% no

Do magazines, influencers and the media make you feel bad about your appearance? – 81% yes 19% no

Those figures are shocking to me, and probably to you too.

I don't have a phd in nutrition. I'm not a therapist. But just like you, I am the 'normal person' who lives in a disordered society. I want to tell you about things that have impacted my recovery and how I'm slowly changing my mindset.

Right now, have a think, what do you want to eat? No food rules, no diet, just go by what your body is wanting right now in this moment. Would you normally eat this? Have a think about when you last ate something you actually enjoyed, rather than what you thought you 'should' eat.

We should not feel guilty about being full, overeating sometimes, getting a second serving, being hungrier than someone else, or anything like that. We are human. We are so deep into this sickening mind-set, that we forget about what 'normal eating' is. Normal eating is going to the table hungry and eating until you are satisfied. It is being able to eat what you feel like. Normal eating is giving thought to your food selection to make sure you get nutrients, but not being so wary and restrictive that you miss out on the enjoyable food. Normal eating is three meals a day, or, four, or five, or munching along the way. It is leaving some biscuits on the plate because you know they will still be there tomorrow, or it is eating all of them because they taste so good. Normal eating is overeating sometimes, feeling stuffed. And it can be undereating at times, wishing that you would have had more. Normal eating is flexible. It changes in response to your hunger, schedule and feelings.

The word 'diet' has become a 'naughty' word, and so the media use the term 'clean eating'. Clean eating is essentially a diet. Food is not clean or dirty. A donut is clean, and so is an apple. The only time I would ever like to hear 'this food is dirty', is when it has literally fallen to the ground and got mud or grit on it. Then, it is dirty.

One thing I cannot reiterate enough is, there is no such thing as 'good' food and 'bad' foods. yes, some foods have better nutrients in them and support the maintenance of your organs and bodily functions, but that doesn't mean they are 'good'. Labelling a food as 'bad' automatically gives us a feeling of guilt or shame, and is a disordered way of thinking about food, yet 'fitness and health influencers' use these terms often, and this terminology has become normal.

Everywhere you look there is some form of diet culture. Look in a magazine and even just on the front page you have a beautiful air brushed woman, and words such as 'lose weight in 7 days', or 'tricks to become perfect'. In adverts you see the perfect couple walking along a beach with sunglasses that will only ever suit them.

There's detoxes to get rid of the pouch on your stomach…where your uterus is. It has come to the point where we are literally body shaming organs. You go to the shops, and there's calorie labels everywhere. You look at a billboard and there's a lean athletic body. My point is, we are constantly being reminded of what we 'should be like'. Most women do not naturally possess the 'ideal' body that we aspire to have. In fact, we have always been happy with our bodies until we were taught not to be. We were never born criticising ourselves.

I currently have a magazine in front of me. These are the words I can see on the front page alone: 'how I healed my skin'; 'immunity tool kit'; 'ultimate abs'; 'food upgrades'; your best body'; 'boost metabolism'. I haven't even opened the magazine and I have been bombarded with diet culture ideas. Thoughts like, 'is my skin okay?', have popped up. This morning I actually looked in the mirror and thought my skin wasn't too bad, but now I'm questioning myself. Imagine what life would be like if magazine front covers shared, 'yummy salad and chocolate cake for the whole family'; 'move your body wisely'; 'you are enough'; 'self-care (that doesn't include detoxes and vitamin drips)'. I know I'd certainly feel more positive and think 'my skin was great this morning, and now I'm going to make a delicious salad for the barbecue and some biscuits or cake'. This fantasy magazine is still promoting health, but in a completely normal, achievable way.

'Summer body'. Those two words earn a lot of money annually. But sod that. If your body looks different than it did last year, it's okay. It is more than okay. You are still you. You are still loved. You are still beautiful. You are enough. You don't need to buy a program to get a bikini body. You already have one, all you need is yourself and a bikini, and there you have it...a bikini body. So, let me just remind you of one thing, or winter body is good enough this summer, and for the whole year. And let's just accept the fact that every female has cellulite. No amount of donkey kicks is going to make stretch marks go, or make cellulite disappear. Something I don't understand is...why do we make it seem so disastrous anyway? Essentially stretch marks are just some lines on our skin, and cellulite is just a few dimples on our butt cheeks. 90% of women and 10% of men have cellulite. We're made to think that it is simply fat, but it is actually not. People of all sizes get cellulite because of fibrous tethers that pull on the fascia that lies underneath your skin, creating a dimpled appearance. Most women get cellulite[2] because of the way our bodies are built; it's to do with hormones and the way male connective tissue is created versus women's. women have higher levels of oestrogen, which fat cells respond to differently than the hormones in males. The older we get, the oestrogen levels rise too, which is why you'll find you don't have cellulite since childhood. Men's connective tissue is also more interwoven than women's. Picture men's connective tissue like mesh on a screen door, it is harder for fat to get through. However, women's connective tissue isn't as tightly formed, therefore leaving more spaces for the fat to get through. (and note this, when I'm talking about fat it doesn't mean you are fat. We are supposed to have fat,

---

[2] Shape. (n.d.). Everything You Ever Wanted to Know About Cellulite. [online] Available at: https://www.shape.com/weight-loss/tips-plans/what-cellulite.

we have fat. We have fingernails but we are not fingernails). Dimples on our cheeks are cute, so why do we hate them so much on our thighs? What is so wrong and tragic about this? Nothing. Absolutely nothing. And that pouch on the bottom of our stomachs that so many want to flatten, is our uterus. We are literally body shaming organs.

Speaking of the uterus and organs...amenorrhoea[3]. This is the loss of the menstrual cycle, which can be caused by stress and low body fat. (this isn't including natural causes of the loss of your period which can be pregnancy, breastfeeding, medicines, PCOS, menopause etc). If you don't have your period, your body isn't producing enough of the important female hormone oestrogen. Due to low oestrogen levels, hormonal imbalances can occur, which can lead to night sweats, insomnia and irritable mood. Low body weight interrupts many hormonal functions in your body, potentially halting ovulation. Excessive exercise is also a factor. Several factors may contribute to this, such as low body fat, stress and high energy expenditure. Mental stress can temporarily alter the functioning of your hypothalamus, which is an area of your brain that controls the hormones that regulate your period. Once your stress decreases, your menstrual cycle should start again. Complications from prolonged loss of your period can result in infertility or osteoporosis. If your body is not producing enough oestrogen, it is unable to maintain

---

[3] Mayoclinic.org. (2019). Amenorrhea - Diagnosis and treatment - Mayo Clinic. [online] Available at: https://www.mayoclinic.org/diseases-conditions/amenorrhea/diagnosis-treatment/drc-20369304.

levels of calcium in your bones, thinning the bone mass. Remember, if you are worried, consult with a doctor.

The University of Glasgow in around 2018 did a study, revealing that just one out of nine bloggers making weight management claims actually provided accurate and trustworthy information. These nine bloggers had over 80.000 followers. The amount of people who have viewed unhelpful information is scary and harmful. Something I ask myself often is, how does Instagram allow this? How does it allow this kind of toxicity and allows advertisement of hunger curbing lolly-pops, yet self-harm scars are being taken down because they are damaging and push people over the edge? That there, is stigma at its finest, but we are so caught up in this mess that we are blinded by reality.

The large growing fitness trend is also causing some concerns. While physical activity and balanced eating is very important, there is a very dark side to it as well. This is orthorexia, an addiction to 'healthy eating and exercise', a strive for 'perfection'. Scientists at the University College London did some research in 2017, finding that the more you use Instagram, the likelier you are to develop orthorexia, especially if you follow 'health and fitness influencers'. Many people, especially young people, are completely obsessed with these public figures, and follow workouts that they post online. The issue with this is the workout may not be right for them and their ability. This either disheartens them and makes them feel weak, or then they get injured. Some of these popular accounts promote happiness, and say they will make you feel better. Be honest with yourself, do they actually make you feel as good as they say they will?

This is something that I experience often, and you may do too. I find that when I go to a food shop and buy loads of fruits and vegetables, the cashier comments on my 'good choices', and when I do a shop filled with chocolate and cake the cashier will say 'you're not eating all that...are you? ooh I see lots of sugar etc'. Personally, I do not need someone to comment on my food choices and make me feel good or bad. Or on holiday I absolutely love the dessert buffet and get two plates, one for watermelon (my favourite), and one filled with cakes. A waiter often looks at me and gives me one of those looks, or may even comment something along the lines of 'are you going to eat all of that sugar? You are greedy'. This should not be normal! These are feeding us negative thoughts, and are completely unnecessary. What should be said is, (maybe don't comment at all), 'enjoy your cakes, they look nice'.

The diet and beauty industry are fast growing, making billions per year. In 2017, the UK State of the Fitness Industry report showed that the business is worth more than £4.7bn annually. Imagine how many businesses would go bust if we started to love ourselves. Imagine how different society would be if instead of spending money getting liposuction, we spent money on charity, family, positive adventures and exciting memories.

Restriction and over exercise have become far too normalised. This encourages body dissatisfaction and negative thinking. How many times have you gone onto Instagram and seen a feed full of tanned, toned women? How many times have you been encouraged to go for a walk rather than watch a film and relax? How many times have you seen posts about 'healthy eating' and 'positive lifestyle changes'? I hate to break the news, but I personally don't think that celery juice is going to be high on my list of things to do to help me be positive and feel better. And if my ankle is sore, I really don't think it's a good idea to listen to influencer Z who tells me my ankle only hurts because I can't be bothered to go for a walk, it's all in the mind she says (and she tells me she's qualified).

Being underweight has more health risks as being overweight, yet we applaud those 'skinny' models and abuse the 'curvy' ones who are in fact happy and healthy. The modelling idea of 'curvy' is actual just the typical body. Where are the 'normal' bodies? Where are the bodies of those who have miraculously carried babies, or battled an illness? Why has it become the norm to only see bodies in the media that for over 80% of women is unattainable? Why are mothers who have just had a baby being pressured into getting back into their old shape and getting back the body 'they lost'? If you're a mum, you have not lost your body. Your body was your child's home for 9 months and brought a new life into this world. Bodies change, they are meant to change. You've grown a human in your stomach, your body is not meant to look as if it hasn't. Get your fitness back, not to show others how you 'bounced back', but to show your children health, to be there for your children when they grow up, and to be able to be the best mum you can be. We have become so used to thinking that thin means healthy and happy, whereas the truth is, it doesn't mean that.

I'm not preaching just eating less nutritious food either. I am preaching balance. And balance is different for everyone. I have chocolate and ice cream, but I also love my fruit and vegetables. I've found that once starting to listen to my body, I actually don't always crave fried food, but I also don't always crave salads. If I want an apple or salad, I will have that, but if I want 3 donuts and ice cream, I will also have that. My balance may be different to yours, and that's ok. You do you, I do me. Health can be determined in so many other ways. How do you feel? How does your body feel? How are your hair and nails? How is your digestion? But to point out, at the beginning of recovering from restriction of any sort, the word 'nutrients' should be put to rest. At the beginning, nutritional value has no importance to you, your goal should be to give your body what it needs, and then you can think about what balance looks like for you.

Research shows that yo-yo dieting damages your metabolism and increases risk of heart disease, high blood pressure, inflammation and loss of muscle. And that's just the physical effects. Psychologically it creates a pattern of disordered eating and behaviours. As if all of this isn't enough, there's the financial strain of memberships, magazines, weight loss equipment, vitamins and 'healthy snacks. You cannot make peace with food if you are still in the diet state of mind.

There was a study[4] in 2004, with 25 most viewed children's programmes, and two thirds of these linked thinness and physical attractiveness with positive personality traits, while 75% of the videos linked

---

[4] HERBOZO, S., TANTLEFF-DUNN, S., GOKEE-LAROSE, J. and THOMPSON, J K. (2004), Beauty and Thinness Messages in Children's Media: A Content Analysis. Eating Disorders, 12(1), pp.21–34.

obesity with unfavourable traits. Then, in 2010, a study[5] showed that 87% of female characters in children's animated programmes were underweight.

This world is consumed in weight loss. But what about weight gain? There are a lot of people who should actually put on a bit more weight rather than lose it. if you're gaining weight in a world that is constantly trying to tell you the opposite, well done, you are bloody amazing. Gaining weight is not 'naughty' or 'criminal', and does not change your worth and beauty.

The effects of diet culture (cheatdaydesign)

2001: 'Healthy option'	Today: 'Foods you think are health but are bad for you'
Fruit smoothie – delicious, healthy and full of vitamins	Fruit smoothie – too much sugar, only drink green vegetable smoothies
Granola – great on-the-go, fibre and protein	Granola – too many calories and sugar, avoid
Yogurt – low cal, yummy snack, full of probiotics	Yogurt – sugary, full of additives. Only eat plain Greek yoghurt.
Eggs – packed with protein and good fats	Eggs – raises your cholesterol
Deli meats – protein packed, easy	Deli meats – processed and packed with too much sodium

---

[5] Northup, T. and Liebler, C.M. (2010). The Good, the Bad, and the Beautiful. Journal of Children and Media, 4(3), pp.265–282.

Now, this is important for those who have been in a restrictive and unhealthy relationship with food, body image and exercise. For those underweight who won't let yourself go over the 'minimum healthy BMI'[6]......
Body mass index. Hundreds of years ago, sure, this was a great way to measure health, but I believe it's time to move on form that. Everybody's healthy is at different weights. Some people are naturally on the slim side, whilst some are naturally healthier at a higher weight. BMI is a measure that used your weight and height to indicate if you are obese, healthy or slim. BMI does not differentiate between fat and muscle, periods, water retention, bone density, time of day, type of scale and so much more. Your health is not defined by a number. You cannot define yourself by just a number, for you are so much more than that. You are the smiles you smile, the laughs you laugh, the hugs you give, the kindness you show others.

How you talk to yourself matters. Too often we downplay ourselves or say negative comments. I've come up with common things that a lot of people say that promotes diet culture, and my task for you is to stop saying them.

1. 'I feel fat'. How about instead of saying that, you say 'I don't feel my best about my body today'.
2. 'you look like you've lost weight'. Even though this may be a compliment you're trying to give someone, have a think about this. Maybe they

---

[6] Roxby, P. (2018). Can we trust BMI to measure obesity? BBC News. [online] 26 Apr. Available at: https://www.bbc.co.uk/news/health-43895508.

lost weight because they have an eating disorder, or an illness, or can't afford food, or lost someone and feel too sick to look after themselves. You never know, you may be feeding someone's eating disorder or pain. However, when someone actually has lost weight in a healthy way, it still shouldn't be the most important thing you say. Try saying, 'you look so much happier, your eyes are glowing, you look beautiful today' instead.

3. 'this food is clean/dirty/guild-free/bad'. Food is food, and should be enjoyed in a healthy way. No food should make you feel guilty. Tell yourself this instead, 'I really fancy some chocolate, so I will have that and satisfy my cravings. Later on, I will have some fruit to get my vitamins in'.

4. 'I'm having a cheat day'. Diet culture police are coming right at you now with their sirens on. Food is not a game! You cannot cheat with food. A cheat meal doesn't exist. It is simply a meal. Diet culture almost makes us need to have a reason to justify why we're eating something, but that shouldn't be necessary. Eat chicken and rice if you fancy that, and eat a burger and chips if you fancy that. You do not need to give an explanation for your food choices, turning them into 'cheat days and meals'.

5. 'you're not fat, you're beautiful'. Well...what about fat *and* beautiful? I think I've said enough about this one.

"Do not let a bit of plastic or glass determine your worth."

Something very common in recovering from disordered eating or an eating disorder is something called *extreme hunger*. In my opinion this is not talked about enough, and is unheard of for so many people.

Let's say I need 3000 calories a day.

That's around 1095000 a year.

Let's say I ate 1000 calories a day for a year. That comes to 365000 a year.

That is a deficit of 730000 calories a year.

Oh wait. I forgot about factoring in the ridiculous amount of exercise I did daily.

Now, even without the deficit form exercise, I have 730000 calories to make up for. No wonder a 900-calorie pizza didn't even make a dent on your hunger.

Over the years of restriction, I created so much deficit that in recovery my mind and body would be so hungry. Unbelievably hungry. Now even though this may not be scientifically complete correct, this is how it is psychologically, and you need to listen to that mental hunger.

It is normal, and you need to listen to it.

It is scary, but the only way to get through extreme hunger is to go through it.

You have got to allow yourself to eat 10,000 calories a day if that's what you need. Its ok, its ok. It's not bingeing, it is normal. Extreme hunger won't last forever, but the more you go against it, the longer it will last. Your hunger will eventually go back to normal, but not until you go through this uncomfortable period first. Not until your body is ready to trust you again. This isn't exactly scientifically proven but it's a growing conversation trend in the recovery community

Your body is in the process of repairing itself, and your body doesn't know when it will get food again, so it sends your mind signals of overwhelming hunger. As you stick with recovery, your body will begin to trust you again, and won't be afraid of not getting food.

"And it's okay if your body feels foreign. Mine did, and sometimes still does. My body sometimes feels like a foreign country. New lines, marks, hills and potholes...a different size and different language. I fled the war zoned country and arrived in a country of peace. I will take time to learn the new language, for here it is love rather than fear and hatred. I still have memories of the war written across my body, and sometime the memories like to consume my mind, or even roll down my cheeks like a stream flowing own a mountain, but they are my history. I am ready to settle in peace and be safe, I'm ready to love my body."

Eating Disorders

Eating disorders are so much more than skipping a few meals and losing weight. They are not something you have on 'the side' while you still enjoy the rest of your life. eating disorders become your life. It is numbers swimming in your mind all day every day. It's the difference between a good day and a bad day just because of 3 calories up or down. Eating disorders are a loss of dignity. It's self-hate, shame and numbness. It is not tragically beautiful; it is a dangerous demon that makes a home in your mind and doesn't want to leave until you're dead. And your job is to try and kill it instead, despite it slowly killing you.

There are many types of eating disorders,[7, 8, 9, 10] such as bingeing, bulimia, diabulimia, orthorexia, EDNOS, anorexia nervosa, atypical anorexia, ARFID and many

[7] Beat. (n.d.). Helplines. [online] Available at: https://www.beateatingdisorders.org.uk/support-services/helplines.

[8] NHS Choices (2019). Eating disorders. [online] NHS. Available at: https://www.nhs.uk/conditions/eating-disorders/.

[9] National Eating Disorders Association. (2018). Warning Signs and Symptoms. [online] Available at: https://www.nationaleatingdisorders.org/warning-signs-and-symptoms.

[10] www.mind.org.uk. (n.d.). Types of eating disorders. [online] Available at: https://www.mind.org.uk/information-support/types-of-mental-health-problems/eating-problems/types of eating-disorders/.

more. However, I am only going to be mainly directing this at those with anorexia tendencies, however the same things apply for the other disorders too in some parts.

'Food isn't going to make me pretty'. Nor are rotten teeth, brittle nails, bruised skin, sunken eyes, hair loss, seizures, fainting...death. Thin does not mean thigh gap. It means legs that can't hold you up anymore. Do you want to know what's better than looking like a model? Looking in the mirror and loving what you see. Disordered eating and eating disorder are not choices. They are serious illnesses and have a deadly death rate. For those suffering, they feel they are never skinny enough, even though they are on deaths door. It's an illness, a murderer. So many people keep it a secret unfortunately, because they're scared. But the truth is, silence can be the biggest killer.'

Anorexia often starts in teenage years and can affect both sexes. I want you to read the bullet points and see how many of these you can relate to or even knew about.

Common thoughts are:
- Negative self-belief and esteem
- Strict rules about food and weight
- A lot of focus on food
- Others are trying to make me fat
- I need to be in control
- I'm worthless
- I need to be healthy
- If I look a certain way then I will be liked

Emotions and illnesses:
- Depression
- Anxiety

- Anger
- Guilt
- Jealousy
- Alcohol and drugs

Behaviours:
- Controlling intake
- Skipping meals
- Hiding food
- Lying about food
- Eating alone
- Cutting up food into small pieces
- Avoiding specific foods
- Vomiting
- Laxative abuse
- Exercising over
- Weighing frequently
- Body checking often
- Isolating and avoiding events especially around food
- Wearing oversized clothes often

They can:
- Make you find concentrating difficult
- Make you tired
- Make you feel ashamed and scared
- Cause issues with education or work
- Stop you from going out with friends and being social
- Cause stomach pain and bloating
- Nausea
- Blood sugar fluctuations
- Blocked intestines
- Constipation

- Sores
- Swelling
- Infections

What to do:
- Seek help
- Exercise plan so not too much done
- Meal plan to eat enough calories daily
- Medication if needed and prescribed
- Avoid magazines or diet related programmes if possible
- Eat with trusted people, not alone S

Dealing with difficult moments:
- Positive self-talk
- Distract yourself with a nice activity
- Be with others
- Write
- Listen to music
- Meditate
- Grounding techniques
- Pamper yourself
- Identify your emotions and see if you can see why you feel that way

"It's ok if you're still on the journey to finding yourself and your happiness. You are amazing, even if right now you don't believe it. don't be afraid to be brave and beautiful, because you deserve love and joy. The more you accept yourself, the better life will seem."

Great things about recovery
- Your fingertips are warm now. What a concept, I know

- Running your hand through your hair and not having hair fall out and get stuck between your fingers
- You have the energy for the little things like reading, colouring, painting, baking, playing with pets
- Liberal use of olive oil
- Not walking a long journey just to get to a shop that sells 'your food'
- Arriving at a restaurant and realising you never even googled the menu

Here are a few general facts that I think are important to know:

- You can have an eating disorder at any weight. I repeat, any weight. Any race, sex, religion and age.
- Australia carried out research which showed that the average recovery time for anorexia nervosa is 8 years
- People with eating disorders may appear healthy yet be extremely ill.
- You do not choose to have an eating disorder. It's not a phase, or for attention, or something that you can just get over with.
- Recovery looks different for everyone. For someone, saying yes to a piece of cake is a recovery win, whereas for someone else saying no would be a recovery win. Don't compare your journey with others, for your is completely unique and individual to you.
- Lots of people who have eating disorders also have depression, anxiety and OCD

- There isn't a 'scale of sickness'. Someone who drowns seven feet is just as dead as someone who drowns twenty feet, remember that.
- For some people, eating disorders are linked to self-harm
- Suicidal thoughts are common with those struggling with food and body image
- Many feel depressed, tired, anxious and dizzy
- Hair becomes dry and may fall out
- Muscles become weak and wasted
- Muscle protein of the heart itself can break down to be used as fuel, weakening the heart.
- Nails become dry and brittle
- Bloating and constipation are common
- Skin becomes dry and scaly, and a fine layer of hair may appear

'We all remember the aching minds and shaking hands, and the monster that stripped us bare. That voice that would soon take over ours, and the pain that became our life. the control that would become uncontrollable, and the identity that we lost to our illness. We all remember how it felt when the mirror became manipulative and the scale was the decider between a good day and a bad day. We all remember the voice that never left us alone, no matter how low our weight would go or how tired and fogged our minds were. The voice that never forgot to remind us that we deserve to punish ourselves and blow out our candles of life. now I just hope that when we remember those horrible, wasted years, we thank whatever it was that drove us from the edge of death. I hope we ow realise that the scales will *never define our worth and can't weight the love inside of you. mirrors can't see into your soul, and the demons will never feed us as much joy as chocolate...the taste of living in a world that we thought we'd never see again'.*

Weight Stigma

Unfortunately, in today's society there is still weight stigma. Weight stigma impacts everyone, especially larger bodies.

In society, we still associate 'fat' with 'unhealthy and lazy'. What shocks me, is that there is actually a higher mortality rate of those who are underweight than overweight. It's just that we're so used to seeing underweight models and slim people that we associate 'health' with it and hear too many stories about 'obesity and diabetes' that we can't seem to understand that although this can be correct in some situations, it's in fact still wrong. You can be overweight but fit, but underweight with no muscles. I think you understand where this is going...

What my point is, is that you need to be healthy for you. Healthy weight for you might be a size 8, or a size 18. As long as you feel good, that's all that really matters, and no one can tell you otherwise.

Thin has become the 'ideal'. Go to the shops, to the park, anywhere. Do you just see the bodies of actresses? Or singers? No, you see a beautiful diversity of shapes and sizes. The media shows us there is only one type of body, whereas in the world there are thousands.

In terms of gaining weight in recovery, ignore everyone. They have no idea what kind of hell you are going through. Lots of people don't understand eating disorders and will still comment on your body, weight and food choices. They may think that they're saying something positive like 'you look healthy' when in fact the eating disorder turns that into 'you look fat'.

Coping with weight gain is something that is important. It is difficult and you do just need to sit with it and be comfortable with being uncomfortable. Perhaps write down reasons to recover and gain weight; donate old smaller clothes to charity shops and buy yourself some lovely new ones; try not to spend too much time looking in the mirror and inspecting your body; write down all the healthy physical changes happening to your body; talk to other people, cry, rant...anything. And after a meal, distract yourself!

Sit with it. Please sit with it. Even though you want to run. Even though it is difficult and heavy. Even though you have no idea how you are going to make it through this. Sit with it, healing happens by feeling.

Where to get help?

I want you to know that help is available. On a daily basis I get messages asking all things periods, recovery and help. Where to get help?

I'm not going to sugar-coat this, but although there is help available, it can be hard to get. There can be 18 month waiting lists or people telling you that you're not sick enough which is complete rubbish.

Here is a list of places you can get help:

- Websites (that also have call numbers and text services) such as: Mind; BeatED; YoungMinds; Samaritans
- GP
- Family, friends, trusted colleague
- In a crisis go to hospital A&E, call 111 or 999
- Therapists and psychologists

For many of you reading this, you may feel like you have to keep your act together and can't admit that you're struggling. But your health is a priority, and you deserve to get the support you need. Don't be afraid to seek support, it doesn't make you weak, in fact it's a very brave thing to do. You deserve the same love and care that you so freely give to others.

"

...as I scrolled through my Instagram, I saw photoshopped images of women with the flattest stomach and most rounded bums. Abs of steel, yet so feminine. Beautiful white smile, silky hair, no cellulite, no marks, just perfection. I saw hundreds of these pictures, and just like many others, I was trapped in the cycle of believing that these pictures were real. I came across a post saying not to eat after 7pm, and so from that day on I decided that it was bad to eat late, and so I started a new regime of eating my last meal earlier. Because if Instagram tells me it will make me fat eating at 7, of course it must be true. Instagram doesn't lie, does it?

By 6.30 I had eaten and brushed my teeth. I lifted my top up and inspected my body in the mirror. I touched my thighs and looked at every inch of my body, listing all the things that were wrong with me.

I looked in the mirror and decided to ask my body what she needed. Less food? Greens? A detox juice? Vitamins and supplements? But my body replied to me and gently whispered, 'please can you just love me like this?'.

My body was telling me that I was enough just as I am. And that I didn't need to change, trying to become something that is not impossible, because those Instagram photos, you see, were fake. Instead of eating plain salad the next day, I ate spinach and pasta in the most delicious creamy sauce. Lots of pasta. And I was happy. I didn't feel guilt, because I had nourished my body and accepted that there are no beauty standards. That I had no need to change myself and look at negativity online. I knew that life was so much more important than the size of your bum.

I learnt to love myself, for the best love is self-love. And the most beautiful bodies are ones that are treated and spoken to with respect and kindness.

"

We talk a lot about how damaging mental health can be for the sufferer, but it is just as painful for the people around that person. I've been both the sufferer, but also the friend, so I know from both sides what it feels like, and from having experienced both, I know that it is really difficult, and it's completely normal for you to feel bad.

You look healthy. And darling, I don't mean you look fat. I mean your face isn't that sickening shade of grey anymore. Your lips aren't cracked and bleeding, and your hair isn't falling out anymore. You seem focused when

I talk to you, and you actually look at me and you listen rather than being unable to stay still or think about anything other than your illness. You seem a lot calmer, stiller, happier, more peaceful and alive. It's easier to have a joke with you now, you even laugh again. There's life about you, I see it in your eyes and your smile. It's in the way you speak and hold yourself up, it's even in your daily tasks. Baby, you look healthy. You look happy. And it really, really suits you. – mother to sick daughter

Here are some things that you should never say:

'You look well. You're looking healthier. It's great to see some colour in your cheeks. You look a little less like you're going to pass out than last month. It's great to have a bit more of you to hug. Good to see you're looking a little less bony'. No, just no.

'You're eating well, which means you're doing better.' – eating better is usually a sign that someone is trying their hardest to get better and this is the first step. They actually may be doing worse mentally because it takes so much strength and courage to eat well.

'I wish I could be as strong as you and lose some weight and look like you.' – there is nothing normal or strong about someone with an eating disorder dieting, and saying this will only make the sufferer think it is normal to lose weight, and encourage them to continue. Being able to starve is not 'strong', it is sick.

'I haven't eaten much today.' – never ever say this, do not talk about how much you have eaten or how little you have eaten. It is extremely triggering.

'Why don't you just eat, it's not that hard?'. – yes, eating disorders are puzzling and it doesn't always make sense as to why someone struggling wouldn't want to nourish their body, but it is not as simple as 'just eating'. If it was, such a large amount of people wouldn't be living with it anymore. Eating sounds so simple, yet it is such a difficult task. And you don't need to point out that there are people in this world without food and make us feel guilty. We already know that, and we feel so guilty already.

'So...are you....do you still...you know...do you still have an eating disorder?' yes, most probably yes. Being at a healthy weight ad eating doesn't mean that the urges aren't there anymore. From the point that someone enters recovery, BeatED research has shown that it takes an average of 3-8 years to be recovered.

'But people don't like it when you're skin and bones' yes, we know. We don't like it either, and anyway, our minds are so distorted that we don't even see them when we look in the mirror...and if they do, they hate it.

'The story is getting a bit old now' we are just as tire of I as you are. We feel guilty and silly for still being stuck in this awful place and it's damaging.

Instead, say these

'I'm not going to leave you. I know I don't understand you fully, but I will try and help you as much as I can. How are you? I like your shoes/necklace/bag. I care about you.'

'I know it's difficult, but I am proud of you' having your struggles acknowledged is so helpful to hear, and knowing that someone understands you are struggling Is comforting.

'It's okay to take a rest day' many sufferers find it difficult to rest, and just let go of all activity for even one day. Sometimes they just need a little reminder that they are allowed to sit and rest, and that nothing will happen to them if they spend the day on the sofa, letting their body heal.

'I believe in you' when someone has lost belief in themselves, having someone believe in them is so powerful.

'Let's do …. Together' it may seem that they don't want to do anything, but that is making their mental health worse to just sit with their thoughts. Do something nice with them, distract them for even just an hour.

Understand that this is not your fault, nor is it the fault of the sufferer. It is nobody's fault. Educate yourself as much as you can about the condition.

Mealtimes can be difficult for everyone, so it's important to try and make it as easy as it can be. Make sure you have everything you need, changes at the last minute can be very stressful. maybe have the radio/tv in the background on. Verbally support them. Talk/be in silence. Have a place mat that's motivational for recovery – this is a good rainy-day activity. If talking, keep the conversations safe

Don't forget to look after yourself…

Although you really want to help someone, it can be upsetting and stressful. You may feel isolated, have less time for yourself, be worried, stressed, anxious, have money worries, lack of sleep, depression, frustration, anger and guilt.

So, to care for yourself, here are some things that you can do.

- Talk about how you feel
- Ask for help if you need it
- Be realistic
- Stay organised
- Find support groups
- take a break and make time for yourself
- Look after your physical health
- Try and sleep as well as you can

I hope when your daughter says that she can't go to school, you listen to her. Please don't tell her that she stayed up too late and it's her fault that she is tired. Instead, push her hair away from her face and look deep into her eyes, and ask her what's wrong. What's bothering her. what's hurting her. Do not rush to work saying feel better from the bottom of the staircase, instead hold her, and stroke her head. I hope when your son's appetite disappears, you notice it. I hope you see his skin go pale, and instead of telling yourself he is stressed and boys can't get eating disorders, you ask him why you can see all of his ribs. I hope you find his blades before he gets sucked into the rut of addiction. If you have scars, I hope you roll back your sleeves and kiss him, telling him the stories he is finally old enough to hear. Don't you dare laugh and say depression only happens to girls. Tell him you have been in the same place than he is, and give him hope. When your daughter rushes home with her girlfriend, smile, and welcome her. When your son grows his hair and wears makeup and tells you he would prefer to be called a girl, tell her she looks great in that skirt. I hope you are proud of your children; they are your little miracles. I hope you love them with all your heart, no matter what their paths lead to.

Exercise

I know we've talked a lot about the effects of exercise in diet culture, but I'm not anti-exercise if it's done properly.

Exercise because it makes you happy. Don't exercise because you are so scared that you ate too much for dinner or because you hate the way your body looks in the mirror. Trust me, loving yourself will get you so much further than hating yourself.

I've decided I'm not going to go back all the way to the days where I was stuck in the disorder, all I will say is I just had a toxic relationship with exercise, so I'll start in August 2019. I had just been discharged, gained weight, and felt lost within myself, but also imbalanced within my body. Before this, I was pretty much sedentary for a couple of months, healing myself. I didn't know who I was or what I wanted to be…I felt like I had lost my identity. But what grabbed me and lit a fire in my soul, was the gym and weights, something that always caught my attention. The first time I stepped in a real gym was when I was around 6, watching my mum finish her exercise. I just remember feeling so intrigued and interested, telling my mum I wanted to go too. She then had to go through the process of telling me that I was too young and could start at 16 if I still wanted to.

It's quite funny to remember how disappointed I was and how 16 seemed so far away.

My whole life before I got sick was focused around being active. As a child my mum took me out every single day to the park, and brought me up outside in the woods walking and breathing in the fresh air. On Sundays we'd go swimming and we'd dance around the house. From the age of 3 I started swimming and dancing, which I absolutely loved. On summer holidays I would choose to do swimming courses and learn new skills, my favourite being the Survival Course, and I danced for a total of 11 years. I've always enjoyed moving my body, it made me smile and proud and happy, and I felt like it was time to start again, this time in the gym. If I was going to find myself, I needed to go back to what gave me life growing up. I also hated the feeling of being physically weak. I had gained a lot of fat and felt completely drained and 'off', and was increasingly tired. I knew the reason why I felt like that, but the challenge was getting those around me to allow me to begin movement again.

I think people around me were definitely sceptical about my decision to get into fitness, especially so soon after my discharge, but I knew that it would be the only thing that would keep me going. I wanted to challenge my mind and body, overcome self-doubt and start living for myself and my passion. So that's exactly what I did, it is the best decision I have ever made and I have not looked back at all.

I had people tell me I'd be sucked back into my disorder, that I was making the wrong decision, slim girls can't lift weights and so on. But I'm the kind of person who wants to prove people wrong, and won't change my mind because someone disagrees with me, so that motivated me even more to start.

I'm not denying that there wasn't a risk, of course there was, but I guess life is one big risk in itself, and in this situation, I had something in my heart that told me it was going to be okay. I felt those words telling me that I need to do it. At the beginning it was also hard as I felt like an alien in the gym, where there were many 'pros' and I could barely lift a 2kg weight. That was, I guess, my first challenge, which I needed. To let go of the fear of what other people think, and not give up because of the fear of being judged. So therefore, I stuck with it, and I have come so far which is unbelievable. It's crazy even to me to think that only a few years ago I couldn't even sit out of bed by myself because my stomach muscles had completely gone, and now I'm able to do hard core exercises and lift weights much heavier than 2kg.

I am fortunate enough to have an amazing personal trainer, who has changed my life. Without him I wouldn't have enough confidence to push myself, and I don't think I would be able to do it healthily either. From lifting 2kg weights and barely managing a press up on my knees, I've moved so far forward. I have been so motivated to eat and continue fuelling my body so I have the energy to exercise and make progress. There is something so empowering about lifting something heavy, and moving onto the next weight, watching myself grow, moving my body and getting into a rhythm and pattern with some of the exercises. On days where I want to relapse, and feel like giving up, this stops me from going back. I've found confidence in myself and a new appreciation for my body. He has been a miracle to me, and I am so grateful to have him as my trainer. In the past 8 months I have come so far and my strength has come so far, and I am absolutely loving it. I am so excited to see where I go in the future. This is only the beginning.

Exercising and eating well for reasons other than losing weight or building huge amounts of muscles really needs to be normalised. I go to relieve stress and help y mental health. I fit into clothes size small still, just about, and numerous times I have been asked if I'm trying to lose weight. No, I've just gained a huge amount of weight thank you very much.

So, now we're going to get a tiny bit more technical. I love to understand my body and mentality towards achieving my goals, and I want you to have a basic understanding as well.

I want you to be aware that please follow your team's plans and care plan for you to keep you safe.

Wellness is made up of physical health, environmental health, spiritual health, intellectual health, social health and emotional health.

The benefits of regular exercise are increased bone mass, improvement of psychological wellbeing, reduces the risk of some diseases. Exercise should be done to improve your quality of life.

Let's have a think about goals. Firstly, establish short term goals. Then think about long- term goals, and make sure that they are realistic. Consider your physical limitations and heredity. You will also want to establish lifetime goals, things you can do to maintain your health that is doable. Once you've thought about these, write them down, and remember these can be changed if necessary.

I now want you to recognise any obstacles that could make reaching your goals more difficult, and understand that some of them will still be priority, for example your children. Learning to create a healthy balance and time for you is very important.

Be aware, that *too much* exercise is just as damaging than too little.

Here's a little body image assessment for you. Perhaps take this test every 3 months and see if you make any progress.

1. I like …….. about my body.

2. I dislike ……… about my body.

3. I find food and eating……….

4. When I look in the mirror, I see………

5. Compared to other I feel my body is………

6. One word to describe my body is……….

Find something that you truly enjoy. If you were to make me cycle, I would really not enjoy it. I've come to the conclusion that the stars and the universe are telling me that cycling isn't for me…I've had two quite funny moments with a bike. One time I rode into a tree, and the other time I rode myself into a lake. And of course, my lovely mum had to jump in to fish me out, covered in algae and leaves and rubbish. So, I think it's safe to say I am not a cyclist. However, someone else may absolutely love it and it brings them power and energy and joy, and it is a really good form of exercise. Someone's sport may be rock climbing, or basketball. I enjoy lifting weights and running, it is my passion, but it may not be yours. And that's okay, there are endless options and paths to go down.

If there's something I want you to get out of this, it's this; I want you to exercise out of self-love, rather than self-hatred.

When I lift a weight above my head, I pretend it's a burden of life. As I use my strength to lift it, my worries are pushed out into the universe. When my muscles ache, I remember that life sometimes hurts too. but when your muscles become stronger and the weight seem lighter, I remember that the hard and heavy times in life wont always seem so hard, as long as you have the determination to keep going.

Hope

My favourite part of this all, is that even after the storm, there is hope. Please know that there is hope. At one point a few years ago, hope wasn't even a word in my dictionary anymore, but I'm pleased to say it has returned. If you are struggling to have hope for yourself, know that I am silently hoping good things for you. I am quietly praying for you to be okay again. Right now, you might say that everything is hopeless, but it's not that there's no hope, it's just that right now hope is hard to find. I hope that you will be happy to be alive, to feel comfortable in your body, and accept yourself. To not be afraid of life and everything that comes with it. To find out who you really are, not what the world tells you to be. I know this book hasn't solved all of your worries, but use this as a guide and reference in your life, and I hope it brings you some comfort. You're not alone, there's millions of warriors like you in this world. Nothing takes more courage than putting yourself back together again, and having courage and hope doesn't me we're not scared or hurting anymore, it simply means that we are stronger than whatever is trying to hurt us. Even when you think you've had enough, you keep going. Scared is what you're feeling, brave is what you're doing. You have so much courage and hope left in you.

Hope is the foundation of recovery. I haven't met anyone in recovery who doesn't have hope. Because the only thing stronger than fear is hope. There can be no recovery without hope. When life hits you and says 'you can't do this' or 'you should just give up', hope whispers 'hang on, you can do this. Things will get better'. Whether we think it or not, hope is a part of everyone's life. We all hope for something. It's built into our brains to believe.

I feel like I've honoured my past self, and also present self, by writing this finally after so many years. The thing about hope is, you don't need to look into the future. Hope is the future. I don't know what the rest of my life will bring, and there are chances of relapse. But what I do know is, I can do this, and I want to live. I don't want to exist or survive anymore; I really want to live. I want to wake up and eat pancakes until I feel satisfied, instead of counting calories, counting the number of pancakes I make so there's enough to feed our hungry stomachs. I want to love, I want to have adventures, I want to feel alive. To be completely real with you, I am terrified of the future and even just thinking about it creates an uncomfortable knot in my stomach. But I've learnt that it's okay to be scared, because it simply means that you're about to do something really, really brave. For me, that brave thing is living.

"Breathe,

You're going to be okay.

Breathe,

You're going to survive this.

Breathe,

You are needed. And loved. You have a place on this earth.

Breathe,

Don't hurt yourself. You deserve so much more than this pain and I'm sorry you're going through such hard times but hold on because there is going to be an end to this. And no, the end is not death.

You tell me that you're hopeless. But that's not true it's just that right now hope is hard to find. But hope will come, it will come.

The end is hope, happiness, life and so much more.

Breathe,

You have so many breaths left."

So, what can you do now to continue improving your wellbeing? Something that works for me is keeping a happy diary. Anything that makes me happy at any moment, whether it's big or small, is quickly written down. Not necessarily a long paragraph, just a few words is enough. Then, in times of doubt, I refer back to that book and read through all the moments I felt at peace, and felt happy. Here are a few examples of things I have written: *'one hour me time with no phone'*; *'filled in a page of my positivity book and thought mindfully'*; *'read some of my book'*; *'I painted my nails and I love how they look'*; *'I got a new pencil case'*.

Learn to get into the habit of thinking about the good, not just the bad. It is so easy to turn a bad moment into a bad day. How many times have you thought 'the weather is so bad it has put me in a bad mood'? I certainly say that a lot. But the fact that the weather is bad shouldn't make us feel like your whole day is ruined. I can assure you, there is still something good in that day, we just need to acknowledge it. However, sometimes it is a bad day. And that's okay. Sometimes no amount of baking, or positive thinking or baths or face masks is going to make you feel better. Allow yourself to feel, feel what you need to feel, but don't let it control you.

'I wish I could give you a list of things to do to love yourself and be happy, but this really isn't a textbook kind of answer. We are so much more than a clothes size, a cup size, or how many followers you have. We are the books we read and the laughs we laugh. The smiles we give the world and the cosy nights in watching your favourite movie on the sofa. We are the things we say and the joy we bring to other people's lives. You are loved for your presence, your strengths, weaknesses, humour, soul and so much more. Do you realise that people love you for so much more than your appearance? We need to learn to have an attitude like that towards ourselves. It's hard, really hard. And some days you hate every inch of yourself and feel stupid and worthless. But those feelings will pass, and your mindset will start developing into one that feeds you sun to grow rather than rain to die'.

Learn to say 'no'. (of course, don't say no in every situation). Have you ever been invited out and said yes, but secretly just wanted a day at home finishing your work and watching the whole series of something really good you found on Netflix? And once you're in that situation you regret saying yes and just want to leave? I have. I think we all have. Maybe your week was bad, you were out the night before, it's your time of the month, or you're just feeling flat. So many of us feel we have to say yes because we have a fear of missing out, or being judged and unliked, being called 'boring'. Please know, that it is perfectly okay to say no and instead lay on the sofa whilst your friends are out and about. Do what you need to do to keep your mental wellbeing as good as it can be, and if that means turning down an invitation, then do that. I know that it's easier said than done, I still say yes more often than I'd like, but it's about consciously realising the mistake, and slowly trying to change. On the other hand, accepting an invite may be better for you. Maybe you're isolating yourself and need to break that cycle. Maybe you don't know what to wear, or what to say and no feels like a way to get out of that anxiety. Like I've said before, it is all about *you*.

Refresh your social media. There are no clean foods, but there is definitely such thing as a clean feed. Unfollow those account that always post their sweaty abs and cauliflower recipes. Unfollow those accounts that feed you negative thoughts and don't serve you any purpose. Instead, follow positive, motivational, body positive, happy accounts, that inspire you and make you feel so much better. You have the control over your social media and who you follow, so choose wisely. Use these platforms in a way that benefits you, not in a way that harms you.

Educate yourself. Use this as a way to get to know yourself, what you enjoy, what your values are. What are you interested in? What brings you joy and passion? It could be: mental health; plants; how the body works; travelling; a certain country; a language; a theory; a religion; a tv show; a person. It could be anything. Take time out of your day to focus on it, it will motivate you, calm you down, make you happy. Personally, I love the human body and how it works during exercise. I'm a 'why' kind of person. I like to know what is making my body stronger, how it scientifically does that, how my body works whilst lifting weights. I have read endless amounts of books on this, watched documentaries and listened to podcasts, and it makes me happy. It has given me a better understanding of myself and I find I can connect to my body in a much deeper and clearer way. So, find your passion, and let that into your life.

"This is to you, the real you. here's to the people who talk others out of suicide but can't do the same for themselves. Here's for those who tell how beautiful people are because they don't want others to feel the way they do. This is for the quiet suicide attempts. The attempts that never existed to anyone else. This is for the attempts that don't have friction burns on your neck and ECG stickers scattered over your body. This is for the 3 am sweat and ache hours after your overdose but it wasn't a 'proper' suicide attempt so you don't do anything about it. you instead just sit there cold, numb and empty, confused for hours and hours being so horribly aware that nobody will ever know about this night, the night you attempted to take your lie, because if It isn't dramatic, then did it really happen?

This is for you, who stay in bed all day with depression. For those who cry on the cold bathroom floor with their head in their hands. For those who drown their feelings in a bottle of pills and alcohol. For those who are always told they're not good enough. For those who feel hopeless. Place your hands on your heart. Can you feel it beating? That's called purpose. Stay alive, please don't hurt yourself. I know it's scary, but it is worth it."

I know you have it in you to get through whatever it is that is going on in your life right now. I want you to believe in yourself. Set yourself free, and start living. Because behind the camera and filters, there is a beautiful world. It's all about the little things. That one time you smiled at yourself instead of cried when you saw your reflection. That moment when you sat down for five minutes and actually felt calm…like really calm. It's about small steps just as much as big steps. Small steps every day is all you need to do, and they can be tiny. Whatever you do, don't stay still, a footstep a day is still going in the right direction, and that's amazing. Some days you will take one step forward, some days eight. It's okay, you're healing.

To be alive is such an incredible thing. To laugh so hard your body forgets to breathe. To scream and eat and see and smell. To be alive is a miracle. It's to have everything. It is so rare, so incredible.

It will be hard. Your unsafe safety net, the one that you know you need to break free from, it feels too dangerous to even think about getting out. But I'll tell you what's even worse, staying in that net and getting tangled up in it. Getting out will be one of the hardest and most exhausting things you will ever have to do, but it will also be the only thing that saves you.

'*I'm not afraid anymore, I'm not going anywhere. I have finally been found after being lost in the dark shadows. I will save myself as I climb up the mountain whilst the ground beneath me crumbles and gives way. The crashing waves will take the weight of my mistakes away. I am so close, there is nothing left to fear. I'm not afraid, and I'm not going anywhere.*'

And remember this, keep your head held high, don't bury your thoughts, because it'll only hit you twice as hard later in life. Your life is precious, please don't sacrifice it. You have survived every single day up until now. Even when you thought you be broken forever, you healed. No matter how hard things have been, you have moved on. I hope you truly believe that you are stronger than whatever is trying to break you.

So, how to be brave? Keep going, no matter what you're going through. Keep swimming, even if you're sure you'd much rather drown. Keep breathing, that is brave. Really brave.

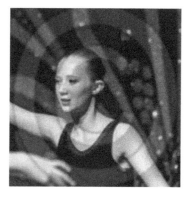
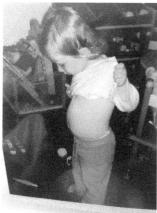
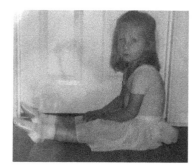
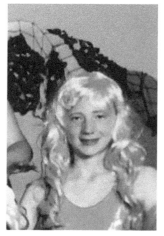

Top left: me in a dance show back in the days when I was dancing up to 6 days a week

Top right: no explanation needed...

Bottom left: starting ballet from a young age

Bottom right: my time to shine as a mermaid in year 6...absolutely stunning

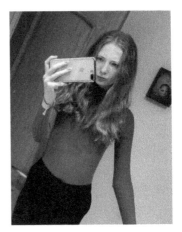

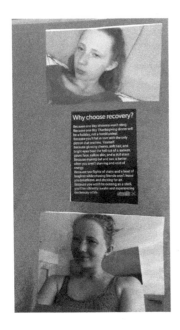

Above: deep in the illness

Left: a comparison between sick and well

Below: my 15th birthday, less than a week before being put on a section 3

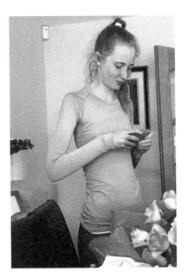

Happy and healthy

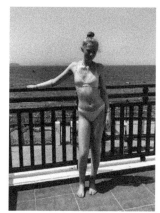
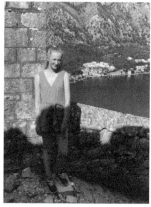

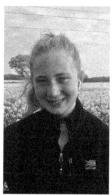

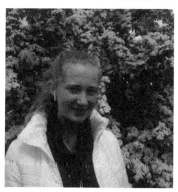
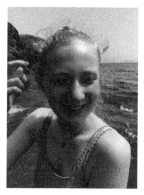

PART THREE

Life is beautiful; you are already so brave

A short story of bravery

Before Admission

It was two in the morning and Abby woke up screaming in a puddle of sweat and tears, her heart beating so fast it felt as if it could have jumped out of her chest. This was just another one of her many nightmares, and once she's up, she's too scared to go back to sleep. She lay there all-night crying, wishing that things would get better. After another long night it was time for her to wake up. Like every day, she woke up at 6.30, heaving herself out of bed, contemplating even getting ready to go to school. It was just another normal Monday morning and Abby felt hopeless. Eventually yes, she did get dressed, but that had used up nearly all of her energy, her mum, who loves her to bits just thought she was tired and being a moody teenager who hated school. She skipped breakfast today, and left home immediately to avoid her mum forcing a banana into her mouth. 'breakfast is very important Abby, it will make you strong to learn', said her mum when she was a little girl. What nobody knew but Abby was, she wasn't a little happy girl anymore, but a teenager who felt worthless and miserable, so scared to go to school that if she did eat, it would all come back up again.

'bitch!'. 'whale!' 'idiot!' 'fat' 'ugly' 'loser'

Every morning during her walk to school she had to try and shield herself from the bullies who threw stones at her, spat at her and verbally abused her. Abby was popular… a popular loner. She'd been humiliated before she'd even stepped foot inside the school. But the abuse didn't stop inside, she'd be laughed and stared at when she walked down the corridor. Alone, with tears building up behind her eyes, she went to hide in the toilets and stayed there until first period. She didn't care if she'd get into trouble for missing form time, nothing could be worse than sitting there alone in the corner watching the time go by. She'd cry, really sob, curled up inside the cubicle. Abby was tired, so tired. And it was so difficult to feel upset and tired when all she wanted to do was feel alive. On some days some of the popular girls would skip assembly to go and do their makeup, and Abby would listen to them gossip about her. some of the things she heard were so hurtful that she had to stuff her jumper in her mouth to prevent her from sobbing and groaning. A few minutes before first period started, she'd re-do her hair and put cold water on her face. She'd take one paracetamol to control her headache caused by crying, and she'd walk out as if nothing had ever happened.

First thing on a Monday morning for Abby was biology, a subject that she actually didn't mind, but the environment ruined it completely for her. Out of all of the topics that they could have been learning, they were doing reproduction, and Abby received hate throughout the entire lesson. She'd get notes thrown to her with drawings and speech bubbles. She'd been called large because of her fully developed body and large breasts. She'd been called a slut because she'd already lost her virginity. She'd been called every horrible thing you could even think of. The sad thing is, Abby truly believed the words that were fed into her daily, and what's even worse is that some of the things were actually true. Abby was mixed race which brought up a whole new level of hatred and racism, but her genetics and culture also meant that she had a body with shape to it. three years before anyone else even wore a bra she had defined breasts, she had strong thighs and a beautiful butt with a slim waist, and she'd started puberty and her period before others. Her skin was the most incredible shade of brown, and in the summer, she'd get freckles on her nose and cheeks which made her glow. She was beautiful, she really was. The comments that were true was that she was no longer a virgin. That was one of Abby's biggest issues in her teenage hood. She had a boyfriend a few months back who was really good looking and was liked by the others. Abby was still questioning her sexuality, for she thought she just fancied boys, but she was beginning to realise that actually she liked both males and females. For a while Abby did question why someone like him would want to be with her, but he seemed so genuine and she was so happy to have someone actually want her, that she just went with it. three months into their relationship they both decided to have sex, and they did. The next morning Abby's face was all over social media and memes had been made about her, and thousands of people knew that she'd had sex. Her boyfriend had said that he had ended the relationship because Abby had forced him to be intimate. It hit her like a wrecking ball, she had been set up to be embarrassed and ashamed. This boy never liked her, but used her. and everyone believed him because they thought that due to her culture, virginity was lost at a younger age than in Europe.

The minute biology had finished she ran out of the classroom and down the corridor, through the doors and down the stairs. Nobody tried to stop her. Nobody even noticed, and the one or two people that did, turned their backs to her. She knew what she had to do. She couldn't take it anymore at school, she just wanted to go home and cry and sleep.

'Baby, what's wrong? You're home early', her mum whispered as she stroked Abby's head.

'I just don't feel very well and the teacher said I could come home to get some rest. I'm going upstairs now, I'll be fine', Abby whispered, just about managing to hold her tears in.

She ran up the stairs, slammed her door shut and curled up under her duvet and slept. She slept for 2 days. Her mum didn't wake her up, but would sit on the edge of her bed every day and look at her daughter sleep, holding her hand during her nightmares. When Abby eventually woke up on Wednesday, Monday just seemed like a blur. She felt rough. Absolutely awful and exhausted, even after so many hours of sleep. She just wanted to sleep again. She didn't want to brush her teeth, shower, do her hair...do anything. Abby's mum knew something was wrong and took her to the GP. What could it be? Chronic fatigue, a heart issue, lack of good nutrition and musical strength? Mental illness didn't even cross her mind. Not because she held a stigma against it, but because she couldn't get herself to believe that her little princess could possibly have a mental illness. She wasn't educated about it either, and that's why she didn't even consider the possibility of Abby suffering from it. At the GP Abby's physical observations were taken and so were her bloods. Her physical health seemed perfect and the results of the blood tests that they received the following week were perfect too. The doctor, Dr Dawn, expected those good results. Even on the first glance of Abby she knew what the problem was. She saw the way Abby's eyes were dark and her hair hadn't been brushed. She noticed the hunched back and the way every step was a heavy thud. Although Abby's mum loved her, she was also very protective, and so Dr Dawn respectfully asked her to leave the room whilst she had a chat with Abby. The conversation ended with the result the Doctor has been expecting. Abby had low self-esteem and depression. Not long after that her mum was brought in and told the diagnosis, and she looked at Abby and said, 'we will get through this together'. As a group the three had decided to put Abby on a waiting list for the mental health services, but since the list was 7 months long, she was prescribed antidepressants and Dr Dawn agreed to see her fortnightly. Sertraline was what Abby was given, 25mg once a day, every day. Her mum had done a lot of research into this, and discovered that sertraline is an SSRI (selective serotonin reuptake inhibitor). Her mum found research from youth mental health charities that suggests that depression or low mood is more likely to occur when the brain does not have enough serotonin, which is a naturally occurring chemical messenger that has a vital role in areas of the brain that control mood and thinking. Therefore, SSRIs are said to work by increasing the levels of serotonin in the brain.

Two weeks later

Abby had been taking her medicine every day for two weeks, and was ready to go to see her doctor and be checked up on. She felt a bit better, perhaps because of the meds, her mum's support or just the fact that she knew what was wrong with her. whatever the reason, she felt better. She felt fine, absolutely perfect. As she sat on the broken chair in the waiting room with a new-born crying and twins arguing over the toy train, and an elderly man coughing continuously, Abby wondered what she was going to tell Dr dawn. Ping! Her name appeared on the screen, telling her that she could go to the clinic room. Although she liked the doctor, she still felt worried and walked to the chair with legs that felt like jelly.

'So, Abby, how are you doing?' asked Dr dawn with a warm smile.

Abby told her the truth, that she felt good and thought that things were really going well. Although the doctor was unsure about how Abby could be so well in just two weeks, her lists of appointments were so long that she felt it was easier to listen to her patient and review her again later. Just like with many other young people, medication seemed to be the 'easy' option and so she sent Abby on her way.

Dr Dawn was looking at her watch, wondering where Abby was. She was usually always on time but thought nothing of it, and expected Abby to come rushing through the doors at any moment laughing, apologising for being late because she was with her friends having fun. Whilst she sat in her room waiting for the young girl to come in, the truth was far from what she was thinking. Ping! She'd received an email and Abby's name caught her attention. In the email there was simply a message, nothing else. 'I don't know how to explain what it feels like to be scared of living and feeling hopeless. This is a way I thought I could describe it. I am having a bath. It is love and warm and peaceful and there's a little candle flickering. It's a happy space and I enjoy my bath, swimming in the warm soapy water feeling weightless. Then I take the plug out, and I don't even think about getting out. Instead I watch the calmness and warmth get sucked into the pipes, leaving me cold and numb. I'm shivering and my relaxing bath isn't so relaxing anymore. Instead of feeling like a weightless mermaid, I'm heavy against the hard tub. The candle is the only thing still there, but even that is just a small flicker of light. That feeling is the closest way I can describe how it feels. I know that I could just get a towel and warm up, but I'm too cold to move, so instead I start to make the tub my home. My cold, lonely and dark home.' Dr Dawn couldn't tell whether to be very impressed with the beautiful piece of writing she'd just read, or if she should be worried.

Two hours before

The world buzzed around Abby. The skies were dark and the air was misty. Faces were blurred and trees became scary shadows. Birds were spying on her and her body felt heavy. Abby had hit rock bottom. She was sitting, curled up in the tunnel under the railway, crying and rocking herself. She had no idea what to do, for she thought things were going so well but now she wanted to escape and be forgotten and lost forever. Not long after that she found herself in Regents Park, collapsed onto a bench so rusty and old that it looked almost as broken as her. 'Miss, you okay?' 'Do you need help?'… the questions kept flooding and voices overlapped each other and the faces all merged into one. 'No!'. Abby yelled no several times, scaring some people away, but leaving a kind looking middle aged woman who was gently talking to her and calming her down. This lady was Maria, and had been clever enough to call an ambulance, but she had a lot more secrets to her, which Abby would find out later. Once the paramedics came, they managed to understand that Abby was in extreme psychological distress and needed help as fast as possible. She was cold and completely out of touch with reality, with a phone full of worried messages and missed phone calls from her mum, who at this point, didn't know who she was. Abby's anxiety was so high and she felt so vulnerable that she thought Maria was a good friend and that they'd been friends for years, refusing to go into the ambulance without her, and so Maria very kindly accompanied Abby to the hospital. 'Incoming psych patient, call the crisis team', said the paramedic to the A&E department. On the journey, Maria opened up about her brother suffering from mental illnesses, which helped Abby feel like she wasn't alone, and that there is hope. Maria and the story of her brother gave her hope and the belief that things would look up for her soon. Once she arrived, her physical observations were taken, and although they weren't perfect, she wasn't in need of physical medical attention, and so she was ready to have an assessment with the crisis psychiatric team. They went through all the usual questions and knew from the very beginning that Abby was not going to go home any time soon. They knew that although there was treatment in the community, she was too far down the waiting list to wait, and the intensive treatment wouldn't be intensive enough for her. their only option was to admit her to the ward and review her again tomorrow to see if after the shock of it all she'd be well enough to go home and be supported there. 'where's my baby?' echoed the whole of the department. Abby's mum had rushed to the hospital in fear and distress, absolutely terrified and ashamed and guilty that she couldn't help her daughter and believed that she was fine today.

The crisis team had found a psychiatric bed for Abby, but would need to wait a couple of days, so in the meantime they decided to admit her and prepare her for the transfer. Abby was in complete denial of being sick and was yelling, shouting that she refused to go into hospital, and so a mental health act assessment was ordered for the next morning. The fact that Abby completely refused to comply with the team meant that they had no other option than to detain her under Section 2 of the mental health act. This meant that Abby, by law, was to be kept in hospital and follow the orders of her team for up to 28 days, and could only be discharged once she was told she was ready. On the section, Abby could not leave hospital whenever, and had little choice in what was happening to her. she was terrified. Abby had no idea what the hospital would be like, what the people would be like, how strict the rules would be…she was scared. Her mum just couldn't stop crying. She felt guilty mostly. Guilty because she thought she failed as a parent, but also guilty because she was happy that she didn't have Abby to deal with when she was in a state like this. The fact that she was relieved that Abby was sectioned hurt her the most, because what loving mother would be relieved that her daughter was going to go to a mental health hospital? But really, what she was most relieved about, was that Abby would be safe and she didn't need to worry every second of every day about her safety anymore.

A few hours before the ambulance would arrive to take Abby to the unit, she got a surprise visit from Dr Dawn, who had been updated after the appointment that Abby was supposed to attend. Her mum had left by this point to go home and pack a suitcase and would take it to the hospital before Abby got there. They wouldn't be allowed to meet until the following day because the staff knew that it would be a distressing time for both of them.

'I'm so sorry you felt that way and I couldn't help you more, but I know you will get through this. And I know you're scared Abby, that's completely normal. You need to get better and for you that means starting your recovery in hospital. I'm always a phone call away, I'll keep in touch with you I promise. Abby, please be brave and strong, you are worthy of this life. I want you to feel like you deserve happiness, the kind that flows through your body. You deserve to know what it feels like to wake up and live rather than wake up and survive. Abby, you deserve to be alive because one of the most tragic things in life is when someone died before they've had the chance to be alive', said the doctor.

Abby had tears streaming down her face, grateful for those words, grateful for a familiar face to bring her some comfort and a peace of mind. The ambulance had arrived, and it was time for the beginning of her journey.

HOSPITAL

Abby was now in the hospital called Sycamore Wood, with fifteen beds. It was old and the walls were a tiring shade of lilac and green, it smelt like an odd scent of warm mould, and the carpet made her head spin in circles. All the doors were locked, some even double locked. The lights were dim, but really yellow, hurting her eyes as she woke up to a woman sitting by her door doing crosswords. She looked up at Abby and with a warm smile introduced herself as a staff member called Elena. Abby hated the idea of being on constant watch, but knew that she had no choice. Elena must have known what she was thinking about and said, 'I know for now you must find it uncomfortable being here, let alone being on a 1:1, but it is for your safety. Don't worry about showering, I will not make you feel scared or self-conscious. Let's go and have a shower, get you ready and take you out to meet the patients, they find it so exciting when a new arrival comes. Reluctantly, Abby removed her clothes and entered the shower, and Elena was at an angle where she could comfortably see Abby but not make her feel scared or angry. By half past eight she was ready to see the unit and the other patients.

'Good morning everyone! Tv down please, we don't need the arguments of Brexit ringing in our ears first thing in the morning. Please welcome our latest admission, Abby. Be kind and welcoming, and have a good day.'

Abby sat down on the sofa and her eyes wandered all around the room. There was a tv with the channel now switched so that it was showing Friends, a coffee table filled with paper, pens, colouring books and card packs. There were around seven other young people and four staff members. One of the staff was sitting by Abby and was her 1:1, another one was also on a 1:1, and the other two were just there to observe and relax for a bit. The first fifteen minutes were extremely awkward. Nobody said a thing and the odd cough or sniff of the nose sounded as if there were microphones in the room. The tension was piercing and the air was warming up, making the silence suffocating. Luckily to break the silence a patient blurted out, 'Hey I'm Skye, I hate awkward silences. Here, most people know why each other ended up here, so what's your story? I have bulimia, anxiety and just a pretty f*cked mind. (at this point a staff member kindly pointed out that she was not to swear). I'm on a section 3 and have already been in for two months. Next to me is Josh, then Max, Nellie, Gem and Olly. We're a good bunch o'kids with messed up minds. Welcome to the dump and we hope you enjoy your stay.'

After that, everyone introduced themselves and gave a deep insight into their stories of how they ended up on the ward. They all seemed nice enough to Abby. A lot of them had turned to alcohol or drugs which upset her, just one more sip for a tortured soul they used to say. Cigarettes kept them occupied. Drugs numbed them. Cutting made them feel. Sex made them feel important, just digging their hearts into an even deeper hole. They took pills to help anxiety. They took pills to make them sleep. They took pills because that was what got them through the day. After everyone's mini speeches Abby spoke. 'Hi Skye and everyone else. I'm Abby, on a section two and I have depression. I've only just been diagnosed recently and honestly things have happened so fast I'm still trying to get my head around this all. I had a bit of an episode...yeah...ummm...and I guess I found myself here.'

Following the little round of introductions everyone got back to reading, drawing, colouring or fiddling around. The day went on and Abby soon got to know the routines and who everyone was.

For the next month Abby was battling her mind. Some days she'd be in a better place, but some days the monsters seemed to possess her and she'd be drugged up by the time the sun set. Although she had weekly therapy, either she was too tired from the medication or just not ready to talk, so instead the focus for a while was on stabilising her mood and then they'd start the 'proper' treatment.

The escape

Week 5

Skye had become Abby's closest friend. For once, Abby had someone who didn't make fun of her ethnicity or body. After a month of being on section Abby had made no progress and was only just being taken off her constant observations, and was therefore put onto a section 3. She got on well with some of the staff and patients, and life inside was getting normal. But Skye...well...they both clicked. They were both on section 3 with no leave, and had similar interests. They cried together, laughed together, wore matching clothes...they were good friends after just two weeks, and by week 5 they were like twins. Skye had dark blue eyes and her hair was dyed beautiful different shades of mermaid colours. Her nose was covered with a few cute freckles, and her voice was calming but strong. You could hear her laugh from the other end of the corridor and it was the most beautiful laugh Abby had ever heard, it was deep and almost earthy. She was struggling, but beautiful. She covered her scarred arms with long sleeves but occasionally Abby saw them if her sleeves lifted up even just a bit. Just like everyone else, she had good days and bad days, but no matter what the day was like, they were always there for each other. In the outside world the two would have probably never met or even thought of being friends, but fate brought them together. In the mornings they'd run to each other and say good morning, sit on the sofa and watch tv together. They'd eat together, sit next to each other in therapy, paint each other's nails and do their hair and tell each other their secrets and struggles. And before they'd go to bed, they'd whisper goodnight to each other, and sometimes slip a little note under their doors. Amongst the pain and terror of being in hospital, their friendship carried them through.

On a long and boring Saturday afternoon after Abby's mum had left, the two girls sat at the end of the corridor by the window, watching the rain trickle down the glass. Abby loved seeing her mum and felt comforted to smell home on her clothes and cuddle into her arms. The unit was quiet, with most patients out on leave and there being a staffing issue. For a rare moment in that building there was silence, and slowly Skye's hand reached over to Abby's. for a moment it felt so normal to Abby that she just held Skye's hand and whispered, 'I really like this. I think I'm falling in love with you'. Skye replied, 'I think I'm falling in love with you too'. Checking that the corridor was clear, they kissed for the first time. From then on to the outside world they were best friends, but their little secret was that they were in love. the hospital rules included not getting into a romantic relationship with patients, but they couldn't help it. they couldn't stop themselves from feeling such intense emotions towards each other. They both knew how risky this was, but they both agreed that they had to try and make to work. They couldn't pretend not to have those feelings even if it broke the rules. Love has no rules, and some rules are meant to be broken.

The next day It was just as quiet as Saturday and the girls had a plan. They were frustrated and tired of not being allowed out after being in hospital for so long and hated seeing other people go out. Today was their escape day. If they weren't allowed the easy way out, they'd go the hard way. It was 10.27 exactly, 3 minutes before the first stage of their plan. The courtyard door was open and they sneaked out, heading towards the fence.

'Oi! What do you think you're doing?', yelled a nurse who had seen them through the window.

The girls had to make something up quickly, they refused to let their plan fail, especially just at the beginning.

'We just want some fresh air and we're so bored, so we've decided to play a childhood game of spies', replied Skye.

'Oh, enjoy then, its lovely to see that you're being creative and thinking back to your childhood. Don't spy on me though!', said the nurse and went back inside with a wink and warm smile.

Without a moment to lose they climbed over the fence before anyone else checked up on them. Thump! They'd landed on the other side of the fence, just missing the stinging nettles and prickly weeds. This was the first time they were outside of the hospital walls in over a month. The voices kept telling them to run away. They knew they weren't safe yet, and ran into the woods that was behind the unit, both knowing the exact route they were going to take. The concentration and sheer determination were so intense that they didn't even say a word to each other until they'd reached their destination, the middle of the woods where there was a little stream, and a path that lead to a railway station and high-street. The moment they got there, they looked at each other and hugged, panting with breathlessness and relief. They couldn't believe that their plan had actually worked, they were free. In the middle of a huge woods with no one else there, they yelled 'freedom!'. They had so much adrenaline and energy and they felt like they were on top of the world. They lay under the night sky and Skye whispered, 'I can't wait to die. I am just so exhausted of trying. So tired of this world'. At that moment Abby felt the edge of her heart start to crack, because she realised that the world could be so very cruel to someone so pure and worthy. She was broken on the floor, crying and crying. Washed out by tiredness, both girls lay next to each other, watching the sunlight force its way through the leaves of the trees towering over them, listening to the quiet trickle of the water flowing in the stream, breaking the deafening silence, which soon sent them to sleep.

'you know...sometimes it feels like nobody understands me and it feels like everyone hates me. I don't think I'd be here if it wasn't for you. I was so done, I was drowning, but then I met you and you saved my life. it feels like we've known each other forever and I trust you so much. You've shown me that it's ok to be myself. I don't need to be ashamed of who I am anymore. Thank you for letting me run to you with your arms wide open. You're so beautiful when you look at me, and I want you to know that you will always be safe with me, I will look after you and you can run to me whenever you need to. If I could, would give you a reason to keep going. I would take away all of your pain if I could, but I can't. I can't even do it for myself. I need you here to fight this war, and this world wouldn't be the same without you. maybe right now you don't believe me, but there will come a time to go, but it's not your time yet. You are so strong Skye. We don't talk about your eating disorder much but I really want you to know that it will never willingly let you go. It will not wake up one morning and tell you that it had fun with you whilst it lasted. It just won't. You are its breath, it's oxygen and life. you are the fuel to its fire. Your eating disorder feeds off of your self-destruction and vulnerability. You could be laying in your grave and it will still tell you that you're not sick enough. Its only intention is to kill you and you can't let that happen. You are really sick, but you are also strong enough to beat it. And I know sleep won't change the tiredness you feel and the stars seemed a lot brighter when you were little, maybe you look up at the night sky and don't see a single star anymore, but you're not alone, the stars are still there. You are never alone and I want you to believe that you can fight this horrible war. You need to keep believing even when all you hear is negativity. In the dark there is a light, you are a warrior. Every time you fall down you get up and rise stronger as the whole damn fire. And I have seen your arms, every single scar is a reminder of a moment when you didn't give in and walked through fire. Please Skye, choose life,' said Abby in the morning. It was so nice to sleep outside, alone in peace with Skye. No response.

Skye was groaning, her head dizzy and her palms sweating. Abby knew well enough that even though it had only been 24hours since Skye took her medication, she was already withdrawing. She also guessed that the previous day Skye hadn't actually taken her meds either. She was rolling around the ground, mumbling words that Abby couldn't make out.

'I think we need to go back, let me get help', said Abby worriedly.

'no, don't you dare. I can't go back there; I want to disappear. Leave me here if you want but I'm tired of trying and I just want this to end. I'm not afraid of the dark', Skye replied with tears in her eyes and pain in her voice.

Abby loved Skye, and because of that she chose not to listen to her and ran for help. She knew that Skye would hate her but she couldn't listen to her. She was too young to die, she had so much life, but she hoped that eventually she would thank her for saving her life. Abby couldn't let her best left and couldn't go yet, she had to hold on. She needed help, she was sick and she did not deserve to die. Skye at this point was completely out of touch with reality and was vomiting up all of the food that she'd eaten, and so Abby ran. She sprinted faster than she thought was possible. She never thought she could feel this way but once she saw the hospital, she felt more relieved than ever. She banged on the front door, screaming, and nurses came running towards her. once they saw the state Abby was in and realised this was an extremely serious situation, the emergency alarm was pulled.

'Go and help Skye. She's dying. Help her. Please!'

Five staff and police were on their way to get Skye, whilst two nurses and a therapist dragged Abby, completely hysterical, to the clinic room, where they lay her down and took her physical observations. After five minutes of calming down as much as she could, she went through the full explanation of what had happened, having panicking attacks, anger attacks and moments of silence every now and then. She thought she'd be in trouble, and although the staff were not happy with her, they were understanding and comforting, knowing that she was sick and that is why she was in hospital in the first place. They were extremely proud of her for running to get help, because she really did save Skye's life. Because of this big incident Abby was put back on 1:1, and was allowed to go to her room for the rest of the day to get herself together a bit more. The staff on her obs were kind enough not to talk about the events that had happened, and instead tried to cheer her up with stories, jokes, films and card games. After all the medication she'd been given, Abby felt fatigued, and nodded off for an afternoon nap. Not long after she'd fallen asleep, she was woken up to someone clearly in distress.

'Get off me. Aaarrrrghhhh. Off. Off. I hate you!'

The screams echoed around the building, sending shivers down Abby's spine. The bangs on the wall vibrated to Abby's bedroom walls. The shrieks could've torn any silence there was and left the rooms shaking and ears ringing. And the moans were a punch in the stomach, going deep into a pit that you wouldn't believe could fit into someone's abdomen. Skye had clearly been found, and she was not doing well. Then...silence. The silence of an IM. Abby's heart ached for Skye, and she felt so many emotions rush through her that she didn't know how to feel anymore, and wanted to sleep and wake up when it was all over.

The rest of the day was spent sleeping and trying to do something a bit more productive in her room, and after even more of the meds she'd been given, she slept throughout the night as well as a baby. She wished she didn't sleep just as well as a baby, she wished she was one. A healthy and happy baby with none of this horror. Luckily the next morning she woke up to Elena giving her a warm smile, who was one of her favourite people in the unit. 'morning angel', she said. 'I heard about your day yesterday, I'm glad you're safe. I know you're worried about Skye, so I'm allowed to tell you that early this morning she was transferred to a securer hospital where she will stay until she is well enough to return back here'. Abby's heart sank, her best friend was gone and she didn't know when she'd be back. She never got to say sorry to Skye or give a final hug, and now she's far away in an even more secure unit. It was hard for Abby to understand this, but Elena continued saying, 'you think we don't know just how close you two are, but trust me, we do. But I hope now that she's gone for a while you realise that you need to save yourself. She's bringing you down when you stick with her, because if she falls down then so do you... she's trying to make you bleed with her. Imagine being seven years old at school in the playground playing stuck in the mud. In recovery you don't want to be stuck in the mud, waiting for someone to save you. because in reality, you are going to have to save yourself. Right now, you're stuck in the mud waiting for Skye to release you, but I want you to understand that recovery doesn't work like that. Let Skye be your friend, let her help you and guide you, but know that you are the one who is going to save you. you see, you can have the best doctors and friends in the world. You can have endless amounts of this and that. It doesn't matter. If you don't want to recovery, you won't. Nobody can make you. nothing is strong enough for that except you. you were once a believer, so start believing again. You know your power, and I know it too. I know the truth seems raw, but it is. Recovery comes from within, the outside is there to help. Let Skye get better, and by the time she's back you can show her how far you've come. Show her your happiness and motivation and let that guide her. I know you also want to save her, but you can't. Be there for her, help her and love her, but she is also the only person who can save her. the secure hospital is just there to keep her alive before she is able to keep herself safe and alive. I know I cannot interfere with your love life, but listen to me when I say that being friends would have worked much better than starting to have a more romantic relationship. Now, let's start fresh today and choose recovery. You've got therapy today and I want you to work on yourself and your wellbeing. Good morning Abby, I hope your flower starts to blossom today.'

Therapy

The room was quiet. The walls were caving in. the blinds were swaying and the clock was ticking. Abby and her therapist were stuck in a bubble and the only way to pop it was for Abby to start opening up.

'So...could you tell me how you're feeling today?', Abby's therapist said, breaking the silence that had powered the little square room.

'What do you think? I'm in this sh*t hole, I'm not going to be happy and loving life, am I?', snapped Abby.

'Ok then. How about this: you tell me what you want to talk about, it can be anything from your favourite ice cream flavour to some of your deepest worries and thoughts. I know you don't want to be here, so why don't we just try and make the best of it, and I will let you have control over these sessions.'

'Fine.'

Silence.

'I don't like myself. I'm not thin or white or rich or beautiful or clever. I'm known as a slut and no one believes me when I say it wasn't my fault. In fact, I hate myself. I have never had to deal with anything more difficult than my own soul. I destroy myself. I tear my skin. It's too dark to see. I destroy myself so that no one else can and I think it's the worst form on control but it is the only kind I know. I'm not brave anymore. I'm trying to hold on but I just can't. I'm so tired. People tell me I am beautiful. I hate it, because beautiful girls do not stand alone in parties or spend hours locked in the school bathroom, or hide in their rooms to cry. Sometimes it feels like a light has been switched off, leaving me alone whilst life moves on. Most days it feels like I am living in my own world, lost in my thoughts. I want to get better, but at the same time I don't. it is scary because we are always told that there is light and hope. It's not that I don't see the light, I do. I see lights and happiness and sunshine and a sparkle in the distance. I struggle to believe that it is hope, because I don't know if it really is a sign of hope and life, or instead fire and death. If I stay here in my dark hole it is safe, or at least safer than going out and facing something that could either save me or kill me.'

Abby said that all in one sentence, not taking a single breath; at the end she sighed out deeply and burst into tears, struggling to catch her breath.

'That's some powerful stuff you've just let out, and if you haven't talked about this to someone, no wonder you're feeling so low. All of this is bottled up in you, and I'm here for you to pour out of it and spill the thoughts to me, and I will help you clean up. I've got an idea that you may like; every week we will look at each aspect of what you just told me, so one week will be body image, then wealth, then race and so on. In time we may realise that they are all connected to each other in some way. How does that sound? It is time to get you back, get you back to being Abby. This is your journey, I'm here to help and guide you.'

'Fine.'

So, every week they discussed in great depth about the issues Abby had raised. There were things that could be connected, and when they did, life made so much more sense. The sessions were tough, intense and over the weeks she would end up going through several boxes of tissues. Some of the memories were painful, but it was in understanding the pain that Abby started to heal.

One day her therapist said something that really resonated with her. she told Abby to imagine a thin person who rarely exercised and abused drugs or alcohol. Whose diet consisted of pizza and burgers and sugary drinks. That person though, was never told that she was disgusting or that her body was unacceptable because they were 'concerned for her health'. The therapist then asked a question to make her think, which was; I'm going to need you to think of a better reason for fatphobia and hatred for anyone who doesn't look like a model because they are probably much healthier than those 'thin' people you see who are in fact extremely unhealthy. And so, whenever the demons of body image whispered 'you're not strong enough to make it through this storm', she whispered back, 'I am the storm'. Abby realised that her body was healthy and happy, and no one could tell her otherwise. She learnt that the world isn't always kind to people who looked like her, even though she looked completely normal. But that was because what the world wants and think is the ideal, isn't actually very normal at all. A big link from this, was how she was blamed for forcing sexual interactions. Of course, a rich popular boy with well-known parents would be the least likely suspect to have sex without the female's consent. Of course, the perfect boy wouldn't 'use' a girl. Once Abby realised that actually she had done nothing wrong and the idiots were the others, she felt like she could begin to move on from that and stop blaming herself. With that huge weight starting to lift off her shoulders, she could now move onto another problem.

Especially after Elena's little speech, Abby's mindset completely switched and people really started to notice her start to come back to life. It was a huge wakeup call and she was motivated to get better, there was a fire and spark inside her that was ready to fight. Yes, every day she still thought about Skye, but in a caring and friendly way. Skye had left Abby in the rain, but instead of drowning she was using this rain to help her grow. Abby was put on new medication which she reacted well to, and was continuing with her therapy sessions and group activities. She made friends with the others but they all liked to keep to themselves which suited Abby completely fine because she was happy to read, write and colour all day long. There were incidents quite often but they became a normal thing for Abby and she bought ear defenders to wear so she really did get some peace and quiet in the lounge. Although time had passed since the absconding and Abby was rarely having incidents, the few incidents she did have were dangerous, and so it was simply safer for her to be kept on constant watch. On her next ward round, however, things changed.

'Hello Abby', said the consultant as she walked into the room where ward round happened. It was quite an intimidating space; there was the consultant, a therapist, a teacher, a ward manager, a staff member and a social worker staring straight at Abby. 'I think we can all agree that you've been here for quite a while now and have progressed in the way that we had hoped, and we think you've had a big breakthrough in the last month or so. We think that it is time to give you a chance to show us what skills you've learnt and that you can manage in the community. As of today, you will be taken off 1:1 and have 2 hours leave every day. If that goes well then next week, I may consider giving you 4 hours leave, and potentially some overnight leaves at home. And Abby... just hold on. You have got a lot of good in you to give, hear me when I say there is more than flesh and bones, and death and darkness. I'm rooting for you, have a good weekend.'

She left the room with sweaty palms and a racing heart, smiling so much her cheeks hurt. Abby couldn't believe the words that had come out of the doctor's mouth. She was thrilled, nervous but thrilled. She was nervous because she hadn't been in the 'outside world' for quite a while and was worried that she wouldn't manage, but she knew that she'd be supported and this was a huge step in recovery and in preparation for her discharge which she hoped would be soon. That afternoon her mum picked her up and gave her a warm smile, excited to finally take Abby out for a while. They decided to go out for lunch to Abby's favourite restaurant to have a well-deserved break from hospital food. As they approached the front doors, anxiety slowly crept in. 'what if I know someone here? What if they look at me? What if I have a breakdown? Am I walking right? Am I holding my head at the right angle?' millions of thoughts were rushing through her mind, and she very nearly decided to go back to the safety of the car, but what gave her some strength was her mum who said, 'I know it's scary, and it's ok. But nobody will look at you, it's simply our favourite restaurant that we've come to ever since you were little. If anything, people should admire you for the incredible amount of strength you've got, your kindness and your determination to recover. Abby, do not be ashamed. Own your body, your mind and your life. Be wonderfully you.' That piece of advice would be something that Abby used for the rest of her life.

Just as planned, leave went well, and Abby continued to progress. 4 months later she was ready to go home, she was ready to be released back into the world, the big, real world. She was so happy; her mum was elated and the staff were so proud. No news had been received about Skye, which worried Abby, but she knew that she couldn't let this get in the way of her recovery. She'd been angry ever since that day, but she sat with that anger long enough until she understood that it was in fact grief.

Abby continued to make progress in the community and was starting to live freely again, seeing friends, getting her education completed, and learning to manage herself. She was really blossoming into something very beautiful and special.

Life after hospital

Abby was now a beautiful young woman. She had just left the stability of her retail assistant job to become a writer. She'd weighed up all the risks and positives, but knew that the risk was worth what the results could be. She had fallen in love with writing ever since the day Skye had gone, using it as a way to cope and deal with life and everything that came with it. she found words so magical, and writing so calming and peaceful, putting all of her feelings down onto the soft white paper, watching the perfectly rounded letters join up. Abby's mind was full of words and books and sentences, creative ideas and passion; she was turning her pain into words, her pain into something beautiful. Most nights you could find herself asleep at her desk, with the little light still on, and a pen by her hand. She'd write and write as if there was no tomorrow, occasionally bringing tea and biscuits to snack on. Right now, she was just living her best life, focused on herself, falling in love with herself, excited about where life was going to take her. She was, for the first time in a very long time, chasing the things that fed her soul and made her happy.

Abby was writing a book dedicated to Skye, who she had not heard from in over a decade. She prayed that Skye was alive and thriving, but that was all she had... hope. She wanted to do something to show her how much she missed her, valued her and loved her, and a book seemed like the best way to honour that. The book was called, 'Life is Beautiful, (How to be Brave when your Friend Disappears)', and her first proof-reader was her boyfriend of 3 years, Jake. They'd met in a coffee shop on a Monday morning. The café was busy and there was one little coffee table left in the corner, Abby and Jake both running for it, dodging people and bags and waitresses and chairs. coincidentally, they reached the table at the same time and had the little awkward conversation of who got there first and the nonsense of 'you sit there...oh no, you sit I didn't even want to sit there'. Luckily, like sensible adults, they decided to share the table and let each other get on with their work silently and independently. For about an hour they completely ignored each other, pretending that they weren't on the same table, but they soon found themselves stuck into a deep conversation and made it a Monday ritual to meet each other at the same café at the same time. By the next couple of weeks, they'd exchanged numbers and were texting often. A few months later, they found themselves deep in love, in awe of each other, and started to date. Jake was special, a rare person with the purest heart possible. He was quiet and introverted which was a trait that Abby loved and connected with. His hazelnut eyes were so warm and soothing, his light brown hair slightly curling when it was getting too long, and a voice so gentle but also so masculine. It was hard for him at first to understand Abby's past, and it took time to learn how to help Abby, but he spent his days researching about mental health, talking to Abby, educating himself, and came to be one of the most supportive and caring people Abby ever knew. He was an artist, creating book covers, children's books illustrations, and was well known, bringing in a steady income. The two lovers were quite a pair, with Jake spending his days in his art studio, the light shining in through the large glass windows, brightening the room, paints and pencils spread out, creating beautiful pieces of art, and Abby lost in her world of words, sitting in her little, dark and cosy room with a yellow light shining over the paper. They then cooked dinner and ate together, going on a daily evening walk down to the lake, where they'd usually just walk in silence, simply taking in the peacefulness and serenity of the outside world. Jake and Abby understood each other well. They didn't need to be on top of each other all day every day, they were happy to be in silence, and liked their own space. But despite that, they were madly in love. for them, it was the little gestures that made their heart flutter, like secretly writing a little note and putting it into their work rooms, or surprising them with flowers picked from the garden, or a surprise dinner. One of the best parts of their relationship was when Jake wrote a note to Abby saying, 'if you're ever scared to tell me something or feeling bad, bring me this note and I will work with you to help you and listen to you'. They made Saturdays a movie night, and the occasional stroke of his hand on her hair, or few seconds of holding hands was all they needed. Abby supported his work, and Jake supported hers. He knew all about Skye and the meaning behind the book, and was even asked to design the cover.

The first page of the book was one of Abby's favourite pages. It wasn't just dedicated to Skye, but it was meaningful to her. it said, *hello life, I am learning more and more to like you again. We've had our highs and lows. We've had gentle winds and scary storms. We've fallen down but risen up. But like trees that lose their leaves in the winter, stripped bare, I did too. I lost my happiness and so much more until I was also stripped bare. But leaves grow back from buds, and flowers blossom when the seasons change. Life, my seasons are changing too. My buds are opening up now, at last, the rain has helped them grow. I'm finding beauty and happiness again, and it's surrounding me, protecting me. Thank you for showing me that despite the cold winters there is still warmth and growth. I have another chance at life.*

The final page was also her favourite, saying *you deserve to know what it feels like to be okay. To feel like this world isn't always against you. to feel like you aren't always treading water just to stop you from drowning. You deserve to be okay. When I say that life gets better, I don't mean that the demons go and your life is all rainbows and sunshine. What I men is, that despite the demons, you're able to enjoy life a little bit more each day. You have a purpose; you want life to keep getting better. There will still be days where you're sure you'd rather eat ice cubes than ice cream, but you don't let the voice get to you. There will still be days where you throw yourself to the hard floor screaming, kicking and hurting. But you didn't self-harm, you kept yourself clean. So, when I say that life gets better, what I really mean is that day by day life seems a little bit brighter and easier to get through. Every single day you're getting stronger, and when the demons get louder and scream, you know they have nearly gone, because you know that things tend to scream when they're dying. Maybe it is not meant to be easy for you. maybe you're one of the rare few who can handle thought times, so keep going and know that things will work out.*

Abby was living, really living now, for she had the two things she always longed for; an outlet for her pain, and someone to love who loved her too. on a Friday evening Abby walked into the kitchen and smiled excitedly, saying to Jake that she'd finally finished her book and was ready to send it to a publisher, which she then did on Saturday morning with the help of her agent. They both waited anxiously, desperate to hear back, worried that the book just wasn't good enough to be published and sent out to the shops around the nation. But they waited, and the unknown soon became known, when Jake heard a screech coming from the hallway. Abby was jumping up and down, crying and laughing, running towards Jake to give him a huge hug...the book was going to be published. Her book, *her* book, was going to be sold in shops all around the country and potentially even translated into other languages to be sold elsewhere. She couldn't believe it was true. There was a time when she didn't even plan on being alive anymore, and saw no future for herself, yet here she was in her own little home with her boyfriend, celebrating the publishing of her first book. When they walked into the bookshop for the first time to see it, it still felt surreal and dreamy. Jake was very good at pointing out to the shoppers that the book was written by 'my beautiful girlfriend', which he liked to say increased the number of books sold.

Months later and Abby's life had changed again. Her book had been an even bigger success than anyone would have ever expected, selling out and getting brilliant reviews from the public, critics and newspapers. She'd written newspaper and magazine articles and been interviewed, opening up and breaking the stigma around mental health. After a while Abby made it clear that she refused to be in the public eye anymore, for her writing was part of her recovery, and was not an act to receive fame. She did get the occasional social media message about how wonderful she was and how she was so inspiring, but after the heat of the few weeks of non-stop publicity, things went back to normal, other than a book signing that would happen a few months later. During all of this, Jake stayed calm and kind and even more in love with Abby, and their relationship continued to grow even stronger. She was even planning her next book about stigma and glorification, which she was still having to face regularly. When she'd go onto Instagram, she'd see memes about mental illness...no harm done...right? She had noticed that there was now this fine line to walk between de-stigmatisation and misuse of mental health terminology. It almost felt as if mental disorders appeared to be compared to eyeshadow palettes, compared and shown around everyone's feeds, black and white images and quotes. In amongst the efforts to reduce the stigma, it had gone too far and was now just romanticising deadly illnesses and symptoms. This angered Abby so much, it hurt her. she needed to write her second book to let all of this sadness and anger out, she couldn't watch society fall deeper into this dark trend.

No rain no flowers

For the first time in a long time, Abby was dipping into a low episode. Her life was cold, freezing her mind that was already growing cold. The thought of death stole her innocence and hope. All of the positivity had worn off and she was left exhausted, confused and overwhelmed. She refused to leave her room, didn't shower for weeks, didn't brush her teeth or hair, and didn't even pick up a pen. She was down in the dumps, in the mud and dirt. On some days she would feel everything and, on some days, she'd feel absolutely nothing. Neither was good, for she couldn't tell if drowning under the waves or dying from the thirst was worse. In fact, Jake and the book signing were the only thing that was just about keeping her going...and her determination to hang on. She knew she wouldn't give up because even if her sun was hiding one day, there was still a chance of light the next day. She would eat no matter how low she felt, because her body had done nothing wrong. She was not going to escape, because even though she had many reasons to run away, she was afraid of getting lost. She was not going to let go, because even though living could be painful, dying would be even more painful.

One evening she wrote; *I want to go back in time and find myself at fifteen. There was one particular moment where I was balanced on the edge of recovery and relapse, trying to decide if I had any reason not to give up and I remember wishing that somebody would just hold me. It did not occur to me to wrap my arms around my own body. Now I have that, and Jake. So, if you're fifteen and with you could stop existing, this is a note form yourself at twenty; it is all going to work out, don't worry.*

That same evening a little slip of paper slid under her door, and it was this letter that saved her this time. *I would one hundred percent rather sit with you for as long you need me to and listen to what you're going through than sit for 15 minutes listening to your eulogy. You are not alone in this; I am here to hold your hand. And keep remembering that sentence your mum told you many years ago. Love Jake xxx*

She got herself together and went to the living room, curling up on next to Jake, and burst into tears. He didn't say anything, but held her and let her cry. He hated to see her in a bad way, but he knew that she needed time to get things in order again. So, time is what he gave her, and time acted like rain. Without the rain there would be no flowers, and without the gift of time, there'd be no happiness. She realised that she was still learning how to go back and reread her chapters without feeling like she wanted to set all of the pages on fire, and that it was ok. Healing takes time, and sometimes the waves are smooth, and occasionally they're rough, and it's ok to feel both. Recovery is a process and the past can sting every now and again when you least expect.

From the next morning she began to get her strength back. On the first day all she did was brush her teeth, but that was a sign that she was coming back to her usual self again. Jake stood by her and supported her, giving her friendly nudges of encouragement, and 3 weeks later Abby was almost out of the little rut. There was almost nothing more beautiful to Jake than seeing her leave the house for the first time in almost a month, in a black dress and beautiful, flowy and flowery kimono. As if this was all planned, the sun shone and created a halo above her head, little bits of pollen floating around like sparkles. He never wanted to forget that moment, and his heart ached with the love that he had for this incredible woman that he was so lucky to call his girlfriend…and hopefully soon to be wife.

Following on from their themes of flowers and growth, they were both going out for an adventure one Sunday morning. Jake had been planning this for quite a few months, anxiously waiting for the day to arrive. He was so afraid of losing Abby and loved her so much that he wanted to be able to call her his wife. They drove a couple of hours to the countryside, their hearts pure and full with love and sunshine. There was nobody around for kilometres, and all they could see was an endless distance of hills and mountains, sheep and cows, and the most beautiful flowers covering the ground like a blanket. Most of that day was spent picnicking and taking in their surroundings and the whirlwind of the past few months. At the top, the warm wind blew against their faces and there was a silence so full of magic. When Abby turned next to face Jake, he was kneeling on one knee with a box in his hands and tears as sparkly as the little diamond on the ring. He choked the words out and without a hesitation, Abby said yes.

If somebody would have been there to film it, it would've looked like a staged scene in a film. They held each other's hands and walked across the fields, Jake placing some wild flowers into Abby's hair. As the sun started to set, they set up their beds for the night, at the top of the hill on the grass. Their camping mattresses were cushioned by the fuzzy grass and they both lay there, holding hands and gazing up at the sky. By the time Jake wanted to say something, Abby had fallen asleep and so he gently covered her with a blanket, kissing her goodnight on her forehead. He just stared at this woman. His fiancé. This strong and powerful girl. Gentle but feisty. The thing about Abby was the magic she held inside her; she could still see the sunset even on the stormiest and darkest days. Not long after that he fell asleep with a smile on his face and the stars remained in his eyes even though they were shut. His mind was the universe and he knew the world was being good to him. Together, they both created a galaxy. their hearts resembled a field of flowers, but their love grew into something science could never explain.

The next morning was cold and foggy so they chose to go home that day rather than stay for another night. They had their first breakfast as an engaged couple sitting under umbrellas in the middle of nowhere, eating freshly cooked sausages that they'd heated over the fire they'd made. It wasn't what they'd planned, but it was absolutely perfect. After they'd downed the last of the sausages and coffee, they packed up all of their things and started their trek to the car.

'Jake, you do know what direction we're meant to be going in don't you?'

'It can't be that hard…we'll find the car.'

'Just admit you have absolutely no idea what way we're supposed to be going. Our phones have no connection and there's nobody around us. Get the bloody map out, I hope you remember your map skills from geography because I don't.'

'Okay okay, calm down. I thought you liked adventures.'

'Well yes, I do…just not these kinds of adventures.'

Jake couldn't help himself from laughing at this point. He had factored everything into this trip except one of the most vital bits, how to find the car. Abby's raging red face set him off even more, and soon even Abby was giggling, even though when Jake pointed it out, she said the wind was tickling her nose. Once they got the map out, they realised that neither of them was particularly good and experienced in this kind of thing.

'Abby give me a hand…this is in a different language I have no idea what I'm looking at.'

'Are you stupid? The map is upside down for goodness sake. I thought you'd at least know which way to hold up a map.'

'You're a genius, it's in English! You never told me you were good at geography.'

Abby couldn't believe how proud he was simply because the map was in English. He acted as if it was the biggest light bulb moment…it was cute, but didn't give her any reassurance that he could actually find the right path back to civilisation. You didn't need to be a geographer to know how to hold a map the right way up. Two hours and three arguments later and they knew exactly what way they needed to go. Their heavy and worn out legs carried them up and down hills, dodging angry wild animals and they almost gave way when they saw the Ford waiting for them just where they'd left it. it was like seeing someone famous, they cheered and were the happiest they'd ever been to see it. It was already the evening by now so they both agreed to extend their little holiday and would sleep the night in the warmth of the car and head home the next morning. Now this was the kind of adventure that Abby liked. Seats down, blankets and snacks, cuddling up in the safety of the cosy car. Their car had a roof that you could see through, and they spent hours looking at constellations and getting deep into astronomical conversations. For the first time ever, Jake opened up about something that meant a lot to him.

'Abby, now seems like the right moment because when I look at the stars, I see my friend. You've shared so much of your life with me, this is something I want ti share with you. it reminds me of you and Skye. The last words my best friend said to me were, I must be gone and live, or stay and die. The scars across his heart were coming to the surface, and although he'd always talked about disappearing, I never believed he would actually do it. one night, I must have been around 16, I found a note on my pillow. There were pages and pages of writing from him. He was the imaginative type of person, speaking in riddles often, so when he wrote that y eyes were as pure as the water, I knew he'd be down at the harbour. That night it was cold. It was dark. The town looked so different at night, and somehow, I kept getting lost despite having lived there my whole life. anyway, soon I could see the reflection of the boats and the moon on the water. I knew exactly where'd he'd be, sitting by the boat of his late father, who had recently died of a fishing accident. As I neared him, he was sobbing, leaning against the wooden post, whispering words I couldn't make out. The first thing I said to her was that it was going to be okay. That's when he lost it. he started yelling at me, saying that he would never be okay. That was the first time I'd seen anyone look so broken. I remember standing there feeling so helpless. One he'd calmed down he said he was going to sail away on the boat into the unknown, trying to find happiness and peace. He said he didn't want to die, he really wants to live, but staying there would end up killing him so he had to go away to be able to continue living. It's been quite a while since he sailed away. He hasn't come back; I haven't heard from him nor do I know if he's okay. But I know he is alive. I see it in the stars and in my heart that he is happy and alive. Don't talk to me about it, I just wanted to let it out.'

After that they lay there in complete silence, the hooting of the owl sending them off to sleep.

Finally, early in the morning they set off on their journey back to the real world. They left home as girlfriend and boyfriend, and now they were returning as husband and wife to be…and a better understanding of each other's map skills. The past few days had really made Abby feel more positive and almost all of the way home she was writing down ideas for her next books, snapping at Jake whenever he jolted the car or tried talking to her. the only thing he was allowed to ask was If she was hungry;

priorities like that were important no matter what she was writing or how concentrated she was. They didn't talk about what Jake had told Abby, but it brought them a sense of trust and ability to say anything without it having to turn into a conversation.

Reunited

A week after the trip it was *the* day. This was Abby's dream finally coming true. She couldn't believe that her book had been so popular and inspirational, and that people wanted to actually meet her and get their books signed. This was what happened to famous authors, and Abby felt like her risks had paid off. Jake was thrilled too, knowing how much this meant to her. He was also pleased for himself, because he had been offered an amazing illustrating job because of the cover he had designed, and this was his dream also coming to life.

Abby sat at the engraved wooden desk professionally, with pens and markers, some water and little bookmarks made by Jack. It was nearly time for the doors to open and for the people to come in. 'this is it', Abby thought. There were people…real people choosing to see her, a single door between her and them. She took a deep breath in, and the doors were opening. Abby knew there'd be people, but she was not expecting it to be so busy and overwhelming. people came flooding in a disorderly fashion, taking pictures of Abby, completely fangirling over her. thankfully the security got them all in order and managed to get everyone queued up. One by one the person would come up to get their book signed, and have a short conversation or take a photo with Abby. Occasionally there'd be a person who really made Abby's heart melt, especially the ones who were brave enough to open up to her about their struggles and how the book has made them reach out. There was one particular girl called Phoebe who told Abby that she had helped her in so many ways. Her best friend had sadly passed a few months back, and she was in pain and deep grief. Abby had inspired her to ask for help, and she was now in therapy receiving support. Although one very precious life had been lost, Phoebe was one less person to make up the statistics. The comments were invaluable, she felt like she had found her purpose. To help people through words.

The day went on and the queue slowly became shorter. Abby had got through 3 pens already and taken hundreds of selfies. This experience had been even better than she was expecting. Being able to really connect with people made her feel like she'd done the right thing and done something good with her life. it made her feel special to know that strangers felt like they could tell her about their lives that probably not even their close friends knew.

There was now only one person left in the queue. Abby was looking down at this point, picking a pen off the floor, and when she finally looked up to greet the final person, she froze. She went half a minute without blinking, just staring at this person. And then she stood up, and gave the biggest hug she had ever given before, tears trickling down her cheeks. Although they hadn't seen each other in years, the connection was there and the similarities were still there.

'Hi', whispered Skye with a slight wobble in her voice and a single teardrop rolling down her cheek.

Abby could not believe what was happening. She was so sure either Skye was dead or even if she was alive, she'd never in a million years read the book. She thought she'd never seen Skye again.

'I've missed you so much. I saw an advert for your book and noticed your name, and so I bought it and ended up reading it in one day. It was amazing, and I cried throughout...you have no idea how much it means to me that you remembered me even after my strange and unexpected exit that night. I want you to know that I have never stopped thinking about you and how you saved my life. you are a wonderful person Abby, and I know this has come as a shock, but I'd like to catch up with you again and start a new friendship.'

Abby was crying happy, emotional tears. 'Oh Skye, I've thought all this time that you were dead. You left so suddenly and all I was told was that you were sent to a securer hospital. I couldn't have left you in the woods to die, I just couldn't. I have thought about you every single day since, and I cannot believe that my book has brought us together again. I've really missed you too, and I have so much to tell you and probably have so much to tell me too. It's been a long day, how about we go outside to the coast and breathe some fresh air, and have a long catch-up.'

They hugged each other and felt the same connection they'd felt so many years before. They knew they would never leave each other again, and would be close friends for the rest of their lives.

A few hours later

Abby and Skye were by the coast, sitting with the wind blowing against their face, and after a few moments of silence, Abby said 'I'm so happy we're alive. We made it'. Skye also said, 'I am sorry about how suddenly I left and how I messed up that day. You saved me, thank you for letting me live to see this day'. And at that moment they both knew that they were going to be okay. That they'd fought their battles and won. They realised that the bravest thing they ever did was to let each other go when they were young and sick, and keep living. Then in silence they just sat smiling, watching the waves peacefully come to the shore and the sun set beautifully on the horizon. What a beautiful thing It is to be alive.

Colour has got me. Colour is in me now. I no longer need to find it and chase after it. it has now got me forever. I know it.

You are strong, brave and beautiful. Never give up, and know that life is worth living no matter how difficult it is.

About the Author

I'm Emilia Adler and I'm 16 from London. I've suffered with mental health issues since 2016 and also have ASD.

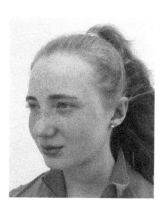

I want to help people and share my story, and my amazing family and friends support me in every way possible.

Lightning Source UK Ltd.
Milton Keynes UK
UKHW050652180722
406001UK00006B/169

9 781839 753671